SEX FROM SCRATCH

For my parents, Marquita and John.
Thank you for not screwing me up.

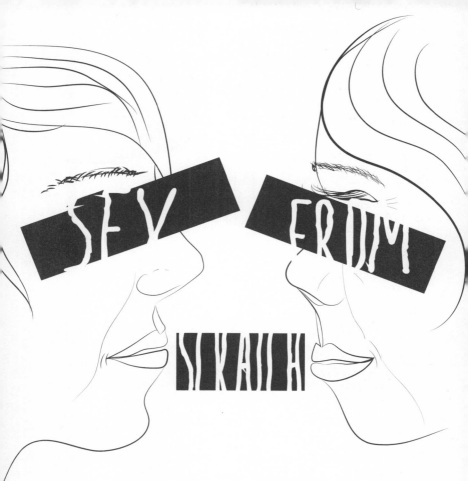

SEX FROM SCRATCH

MAKING YOUR OWN RELATIONSHIP RULES

SARAH MIRK

Sex From Scratch
Making Your Own Relationship Rules

Sarah Mirk

First printing, August 1, 2014
All text is © Sarah Mirk, 2014
This edition is © by Microcosm Publishing, 2014

Microcosm Publishing
2752 N Williams Ave
Portland, OR 97227

In the Real World series

For a catalog, write or visit
MicrocosmPublishing.com

ISBN 978-1-934620-13-7
This is Microcosm #155

Edited by Joe Biel, Lauren Hage, and Erik Spellmeyer
Designed by Joe Biel
Cover by Meggyn Pommerleau
Portraits and street scenes illustrated by Natalie Nourigat. Quotes illustrated by Molly Schaeffer.

Distributed in the United States and Canada by Independent Publishers Group and in Europe by Turnaround.

This book was printed on post-consumer paper by union workers in the United States.

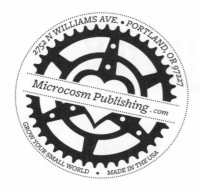

*I choose to love   this time   for once
with all my intelligence*

—Adrienne Rich

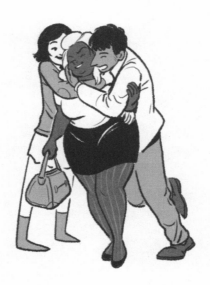

TABLE OF CONTENTS

Introduction

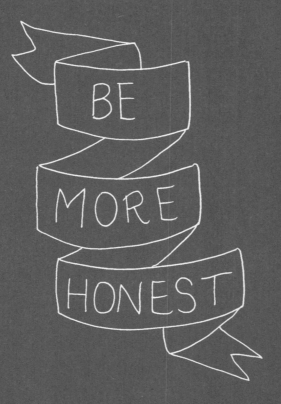

BE

MORE

HONEST

Look, I don't know what I'm doing.

Most advice books are written by people who say they're experts and they sell you on the notion that there are secrets inside that will transform your life. I have to tell you some bad news: I'm no expert. There are no secrets here. Only you can change your life. Sorry.

What is in this book is a bunch of good insights, practical advice, and admissions of honest mistakes from people who are not selling anything except the idea that everyone should feel empowered to have a healthy and happy romantic life that looks however they want it to. It's a do-it-yourself approach to relationships and it's a hard road, that's for sure.

When I hit my mid-twenties in a long-term relationship that didn't feel quite right, I didn't know where to turn. My boyfriend Carl was great. He's funny, he's generous, he's the smartest person I know. But I wasn't certain whether I wanted to keep dating him, whether I wanted to get married and have kids with him, and have sex with only him forever. It felt like the world was closing down a bit when I thought about that, but I wasn't sure why.

I was raised by open-minded parents in the feel-good early nineties, and was taught to have a clear vision of who I am, encouraged to "just be myself" by every TV special since 1986. We're told over and over to be proud of our differences and embrace all of our own quirks. But when it comes to relationships with *other* people, our role models don't encourage quite so much originality. Instead, our vision of dating is very straightforward: No matter what kind of weirdo you are, you aspire to someday get married, you aspire to have kids, you actively work to have sex with one person for most of your life, and whoever's relationship lasts the longest wins. As I started to evaluate whether my relationship was healthy for me, I started to realize that though I knew a lot about myself, I didn't know a lot about how I wanted to be in a relationships with other people. I started recognizing that a lot of what I grew up learning about relationships is based on religions that I don't believe in and on old-school ways of thinking that come from generations long before mine. Part of why I felt so lost is because I had no value set for relationships that felt honest and relevant to me.

It's not just me. In America, fewer people than ever identify with any specific religion. People are getting married later than ever, or not at all. More and more people feel comfortable identifying as queer and genderqueer. The rigid traditional benchmarks of success—marriage, monogamy, and kids—aren't useful for everyone. When people try to squeeze their relationships and identities into that vision, they often find that it's an awkward, unhealthy, and destructive fit. We need a better understanding of what a "successful" relationship looks like.

I worked as a newspaper reporter for years and I know that in reporting, you rarely rely on just one person's perspective. Instead, the most honest stories usually come from analyzing a diversity of experiences. When trying to make decisions about my own relationships, I was anxious that basing my romantic choices on only my limited experience and narrow perspective would inevitably mean making terrible mistakes and breaking the hearts of people I love, over and over. Or, maybe worse, I'd wind up trapped in a relationship that slowly drives me crazy over time.

One winter, on a Friday, after I got off work writing at the newspaper, I visited the relationship section of a bookstore, looking for some kind of guidance. The dating section of the bookstore during Friday happy hour is a weird scene. But I avoided eye contact and focused on the books. I didn't find much. Almost all the books about relationships are specifically focused on trying to snag a man and get married to him. I don't think that goal-oriented approach to relationships sounds like a good idea, plus I'm not so into competitive sports. A couple other books—like *The Ethical Slut*, *Opening Up*, and others mentioned in the endnotes of this book—offered refreshing alternative visions of relationships. But they were all pretty focused on one specific type of relationship and I wasn't sure what kind of relationship was good for me. I wasn't certain what I wanted at all.

I wanted to find a book on the relationship shelf that would gather the collective wisdom of what people older, wiser, and braver than myself had learned. I wanted to read about people who have learned the hard way. That book didn't exist, so I decided to write it.

I spent the next two years interviewing nearly 100 people around the United States about their relationships as well as charting my own experiences. Since so many people trusted their darkest thoughts and mistakes to me, I feel that I have an obligation to put myself on the line and get vulnerable as well.

During the time that I researched this book, Carl and I went through ups and downs. We talked about our relationship a lot. We had many hilarious adventures. I stole his sweaters. He fixed my bike. All the things I discussed with strangers about relationships were put into personal practice as we tried to build the most healthy, fun, loving, and equitable relationship we could. We could be brutally honest with each other—I told him things about myself and my fears that I had never planned to. In the end, we decided to break up. It was slow and it was good. I moved out, we saw a counselor. Finally, we talked and cried in a park right next to where someone had graffitied that line of '80s movie wisdom: "Be Excellent to Each Other." We were. And now we're great friends.

In the meantime, I slept on sofas in Seattle, Vancouver BC, Portland, San Francisco, Los Angeles, Madison, New York City, and Boston, and interviewed people in Iowa, Illinois, Idaho, Virginia, Missouri, and all over New England on the phone. I met up with friends-of-friends in coffee shops, recorded heart-to-hearts with old friends over sandwiches, and, one time, a group of strangers in Jamaica Plains hosted a polyamory potluck in my honor.

This was research I funded myself because I was curious, and let me clearly stress that it was not scientific. It's anecdotal. The focus of this book is very narrow in some ways, being almost entirely about Americans, and is undoubtedly biased by my perspective as a straight, white woman who was raised middle-class. Almost every one of the people I talked to were over the age of 25 and only a few were in their 50s and older. Most of them were white—about a quarter were people of color. Many were spiritual or religious but only a few were practicing. Most identified as either male or female and most identified as straight, though about 30 percent were queer and ten percent were transgender or genderqueer.

I didn't collect quantitative statistics on how often specific demographics get divorced or the average age at which someone typically realizes that everything they know is wrong. Instead, I focused on the stories about people's lived experiences that I hope can act as examples for how to be intentional about the life you build.

Each chapter focuses on a specific type of relationship or identity. Because I like to keep things easy to read, each chapter includes a list of lessons. The end of each chapter includes extended interviews with people who were brave enough to put their names in a book about sex and dating. You can read the whole book through or you can pick and choose the chapters you think sound most interesting. Every chapter is relevant to all sorts of people, whether or not you want the kind of relationship described. That's the whole idea—we have a lot to learn from people.

What's exciting about the relationships featured in this book is that they show the many opportunities we have, being alive today. Though our rights and abilities are limited by politics, economics, and discrimination of various stripes, we live in a time in America where many women no longer need to get married to be financially stable, where we have the technology to control whether we want to have kids, and where we're able to protect ourselves rather reliably against sexually transmitted diseases.

There are plenty of perspectives and types of relationships this book leaves out. The big caveat to the ideas discussed here is that they all apply to relationships that have a baseline level of safety and mutual respect. Most of the advice for having healthy and happy relationships doesn't apply to relationships that are physically or emotionally abusive. The skills and ideas here are meant to help people have better and more honest *consensual* relationships. Building a culture that makes it easier to avoid and recognize abusive relationships and end rape is an essential field of study—but it's not the focus of this project.

This book does not deeply cover bondage, dominance, sadism, and masochism (BDSM) or much discussion of celibacy. I interviewed a number of people who are into BDSM and thought it would be better to incorporate their experiences throughout the book rather than having a special chapter just about BDSM. I originally planned on having a chapter about celibate relationships, including people who identify as asexual. But when I sat down to write it, the chapter just didn't feel right. Everyone I spoke with had very different reasons for not having sex in their relationships, from people who had experienced major trauma and didn't feel comfortable having sex for a long time, to people who feel comfortable with their sexuality and bodies but have an extremely low sex drive. Among asexual folks, people experience their asexuality so differently that there were few patterns or big ideas that I could write a cohesive and distinct chapter around. Instead, people who aren't having sex in their relationships were applying the same critical thinking to their dating lives in all sorts of relationships: being intentional, figuring out what they want and need, and talking honestly with partners. From the folks who identify as asexual, the only lesson that I kept hearing again and again is that asexuality is real, sex drive varies on a spectrum, and relationships without intercourse are still valid and loving. Instead of writing a chapter, it seemed like I should just type one line: *Asexuality is real and valid.*

So there we go.

Every day, many people around the country are making decisions about how they will be happiest, healthiest, and most honest with themselves and their romantic partners. Whether it's making the decision to get married, the decision to get divorced, the decision to sleep around, or the decision to be monogamous.

Let's create an ethical framework for romantic relationships not built on religion or tradition. There is no destiny in relationships; we make our lives for ourselves. The advice in here is for all kinds of people in different types of relationships, including people—like me—who think they'll probably someday decide to get married, be monogamous and have kids, and people who are already doing those things and also people who think all of that sounds like a horrible idea.

There are no universally right decisions to make in building good relationships. Instead, what's important is to understand that there *are* decisions to make and to be intentional about making them. Regardless of the narrow image of sex and dating we see on TV and in films, there are many viable ways to be in a healthy relationship. Given a certain level of economic, political, and social privilege, we have the ability to make our relationships look however we want.

So even though there is no check-off list of sure-fire secrets to happy marriage or must-know tricks to obtain a perfect love life, there are personal skills and ways of thinking critically that can help any person have healthier relationships. It's a hard and honest way but, oh man, it's a lot more fun.

1.

Loving
Being
Single

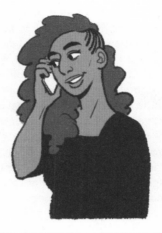

Unlike most of the relationships in this book, everyone knows what it's like to be single. I certainly do.

We think of being single as a problem. Our culture enforces the idea that we should have a little bit of time being single (freshman year of college! Woo!) but the goal is to end singledom as quickly as possible. Let's consider the opposite approach: to relax into being single. Instead of seeing being single as an unfortunate malady that we must remedy, being single is useful. Having a long-term partner can greatly add to your life, of course, but being single can hone some serious skills. If we do wind up in committed, long-term relationships, it's useful to carry over into all of our relationships the skills we learn as we're spending time on our own. The ideas in this chapter are both for people who are currently single and a reminder to folks in relationships that there is a lot to learn from people who are fabulously negotiating the gray area.

When I'm dating someone long-term, I romanticize what it was like to not have my life entwined with someone else. I'd have so much independence! I would read so many books! Maybe even exercise! I'd date so many cuties! But then in the morning, when my boyfriend and I wake up together, warm and with our feet piling on top of each other like they always do, my memories of being single all turn gross and melancholy. I was so alone! I sent so many questionable text messages!

For a long time, my reference point for being single was when my college boyfriend and I broke up. We dated from when I was fresh out of high school all the way to our senior year in college and when we split, my sorrow was strong. Mixed in to the general sadness of letting go of our relationship was some loneliness and some fearlessness. I was single! What did it *mean*? There's a real narrative that if you're single, you've got to be unhappy about it. How many movies are there that end with the main character being happily single? You know who's single? Jon Arbuckle from Garfield. And various serial killers. Being single conjures up images of dark nights and half-eaten pints of Ben and Jerry's.

In my best moments as a single person, I really do value my independence, read great books, get exercise, and have fun dating. After going through a scary, heartwrenching break up, asking out guys I don't know well seems easy. What's the worst that could happen? Let's make out, already. We've got no baggage together. It's all so simple.

But my devil-may-care attitude is always edged with a will-he-call-me-back hopefulness. I get a little tender, no matter what. Our language around dating forces people into a binary situation: are you single? Or do you have a girlfriend? We all know it's more complicated than that.

A lot of dating exists in that grey area between dating-and-not-dating. As a single person, sometimes it's a lot of fun to not really be certain about whether you'll kiss someone at the end of the night. But uncertainty around boundaries, intentions, and expectations also leads to anxiety, awkwardness, and questions around consent. How do we get more of the fun of being single—the independence, the great connections with new people, the good personal habits—and less of the rough stuff—the loneliness, the fear of getting hurt, the frustrating ambiguity? I never really want to be "casual" about dating people; that makes it seem like I just wind up with people by accident. I want to be intentional, but with not a lot of expectations.

Being happy, healthy, and single has always required the support of my friends, through both the fearless moments and the lonely times. Being single, I invest more in friends. We have those dark conversations and share those low, real, insecure times; we have those nights of sweaty dancing and summer outrageousness.

I find being single very useful—it helps me develop a network of beloved people I trust, rather than relying on just one partner. It helps me focus more on the life I want to build on my own. It's helps me learn about what I rely on partners for emotionally. It helps me have more frank and honest conversations with people I go on dates with, since we're starting from a clean slate.

The Details
No relationship is clean cut. But when you're single, things are always a little ambiguous. Maybe you're going on dates, maybe you're not. Maybe you're taking time to be alone, maybe you're just not wanting to waste time with people you don't want to be with long-term. Maybe you want to be single, maybe you're constantly wishing you weren't single. Whatever the case, it's a good situation for figuring out what you really want—to put it in purely analytical terms, I see it as a time for collecting data points on what feels good and healthy. When you're single, it's sometimes easier to explore what you like and want. You hypothetically start fresh with each date and can establish whatever kind of communication you want. Of course, it's not that rosy—it's scary to be single, sometimes, as you open up to new people and realize all the baggage you're still hauling around.

As the phrase goes, "Wherever you go, there you are." Sometimes it's very nice to recognize who you are. Sometimes, let's be honest, it's a disappointing revelation.

Sixteen Lessons From People Who Are Single
1. **Be nice to each other.**
   So much advice about dating is essentially about trying to manipulate someone into dating you. But this isn't a game. It's certainly not about conquest or winning. It's learning about yourself, learning about other humans, and having fun. A good baseline to start with is "be nice." Twenty-something musician Patrick has one basic rule for dating and it's to respect one another. I like that. Start by respecting yourself and valuing what's good about you.
2. **Build a life you love.**
   Being single can be a great opportunity to focus on yourself. I am personally physically healthier when I'm

single—I actually exercise. A lot of people choose to be single for periods of time to focus on personal work, like their job or getting mentally healthy. Women, especially, are taught to define themselves by their partner. That's unhealthy. It's easy to feel pressured into dating people and having sex because society values that over being by ourselves. Instead, only date people if you really want to. Take time to build a life you love for yourself. "Feeling good about loving other people is much easier when you love yourself," says middle-aged San Francisco mom Ellen, who only learned that lesson through therapy. She recommends you don't chase after anyone for a long time, but make a life that other people feel good about being a part of.

3. **Your identity doesn't hinge on whom you date.**
We see being single as being a problem. Though it's not ideal long-term for many people, it's certainly a fine way to be for a while. It's easy to slip into fixating on one person or (more typically) the idea of a person as a way to solve all our problems. "I'd be so much happier, if only Chris would be my girlfriend!" It *is* definitely nice to have great people to date, but it's not so healthy to see dating people as a solution to specific problems in life.

4. **Date people who add to your life.**
This is advice from my mom. It can feel cool to be asked out and it's fun to flirt with people, but what matters most is that you feel good. Dating people who you don't respect will only lead to violating rule number one above. Chicago native Tiffany thinks of dating like a bookstore. You're not going to waste time reading boring books, when there are so many great ones you're never going to have time to read. Being single is a great opportunity to date some of the wildly diverse array of interesting people in the world. And to stop dating them, too, when you decide the time is right.

5. **Romantic partners are not always sexual partners.**
Feel empowered to work out whatever arrangement you want with people you're dating. It's rare to be with someone that you connect with romantically, sexually, on deep values, and as a friend. Instead, value the connections you have for what they are. Engineer

Sarah, 27, had a couple different relationships going when we talked. She was single, but going on dates once a week or so with a regular guy with whom she had sex. Also about once a week, she would hang out with a guy with whom she only made out. On top of that, she had a "cozy friend"—a guy with whom she often just made dinner and fell asleep with. All of these are partners of some kind—she has good, lengthy conversations with all of them and is attracted to all of them—but though they do sweet things for each other, they're not necessarily romantic and none of them expects to be her "boyfriend."

6. **Everyone loves a great appreciator.**
   Sometimes it can feel scarier to say something sincerely nice about someone than to get naked. Isn't that ridiculous? Being an appreciator is looked down upon, but it's a great skill. We all have weird issues with our bodies and identities, so part of being respectful in dating new people is making it safe for people to feel comfortable about themselves. Respectful musician Patrick finds that the best way to do this is through genuine compliments. Saying, "You look beautiful" or "I really like your body" can go a long way toward helping new partners feel less anxious.

7. **Getting vulnerable is terrifying.** Dating opens a can of worms. Even if people seem totally comfortable and casual, you never know what kind of land mines people have when they start to flirt and get physical. Or what land mines you have yourself, frankly. Since we don't come equipped with simple road maps, the best we can do is recognize that keeping close to someone— whether it's sexual or just as a friend—can dig up parts of ourselves we try to avoid. Feeling okay with being sexual is a lot easier for some people than others, so take your time, be patient, and keep talking. It's worthwhile to keep some armor on, so to speak, and watch out for yourself when you're single—building trust takes time and learning about one another.

8. **Get intentional.**
   Human history proves that the most sure-fire way to make enemies is to be a sloppy dater. Even casual sex should be intentional. It's fun to ask someone out

on a whim or kiss them on the spur of the moment, but the aforementioned emotional land mines are no joke. Pay attention to how you both are feeling and talk about boundaries. You really can have whatever kind of relationship you want with someone in that gray area between "just friends" and "boyfriend/girlfriend"—having sex, not having sex, just being cuddly—as long as you're intentional about what you're doing. Sarah, the engineer who is dating multiple guys, has had conversations with each of them about her intentions. She's told them all that she doesn't want to be monogamous and doesn't expect any of them to be her boyfriend. In the moment, they discuss one-on-one how they feel and how far they want to go physically. Things go much more smoothly and everyone knows where they stand now that they're all on the same page.

9. **Make a move, if you want to.**

   I've talked to so many straight women who lament the amount of time they waste waiting for a guy to make a move. This seems like a mostly heterosexual problem, for some reason, one that's rooted in puritanical ideas that if women express desire, they're "coming on too strong" and being slutty. Screw that. If you want to ask a guy out, straight women, ask him out! Same goes for the straight guys. The key here is being respectful in the way you ask; bring it up only if the idea seems appropriate, and you're ready to accept possible rejection without awkwardness.

10. **Only exchange bodily fluids with people you trust.**

    Okay, I know this is not a very catchy slogan, but it's far more accurate than "don't sleep with anyone until the third date." Have sex with people whenever you want to, but recognize that the stakes are high. If you don't feel comfortable enough with someone to ask them the date of their most recent STD test and, if it's hetero sex, to discuss what birth control method you're going to use, *don't have sex*. Having sex requires a basic conversation.

11. **Safer sex takes work.**

    So much work! This goes for people in non-monogamous relationships, too, but if you're single and dating numerous new people, it can be a constant workflow.

Get tested for STDs at least every six months if you're having sex with people and insist that your partners do too. Talk with partners about their sexual health and make time to talk about and know those land mines that can relate to history and insecurities. It means being active about consent.

12. **Don't get consent through telepathy.**

Attempting to discern the sexual desires and limits of a new partner via transmission of mental brainwaves will only lead to trouble. So will expressing your own wants and needs through purely nonverbal clues. Ask—out loud—whether it's okay to get physical. "Can I kiss you?" is one of the sexiest phrases in the English language. "I'm really attracted to you, but let's take it slow—I don't want to have sex tonight" is pretty hot, too. Of course, consent is the basis of any sexy relationship. But it comes up especially when people who don't know each other well—and who are probably still trying to impress each other and seem cool—start getting it on. In movies, lovers just *know*. In real life, it's never okay to assume that because someone invited you to dinner that they'll want to make out or that because you're in bed that they want to have sex.

13. **Skip blurred lines—being direct is sexy.**

When a date gets on into the evening, musician and bike-builder Travis always tries to clearly tell partners what he wants, saying something like, "I'd really like you to sleep over, but I don't want to have sex." But what "sex" means, of course, varies by the person, so that kind of statement is only a good starting point for conversation that happens throughout the evening. This doesn't mean you need to launch into a soliloquy listing every single way you like to be touched, but many people say that guidance and clear limits help them feel at ease. Travis says he feels much more comfortable with partners who can tell him what they like and don't like. When a guy tells him they like having their neck kissed or a girl says she doesn't like her nipples nibbled quite so hard, that's helpful feedback he can use to be a better lover.

14. Talk about your expectations.

What does it mean to be hooking up? Are you on the tenure-track to a long-term partner situation or do you just want to take each day as it comes? When graphic designer Molly started dating a cute guy from her yoga class, before they had sex, they talked about how they didn't want to develop "feelings" for each other—meaning, in their case, that neither wanted to fall in love.

15. Don't go radio silent.

Charlie, an artist in Seattle, was dating a girl kind of seriously—they'd hung out a couple nights a week for more than a month, were having sex—and then she just stopped calling him back. She stopped replying to his texts. Without a conversation about what was going right or wrong, she dropped off the map. My friends call this phenomena "going radio silent" and it is infuriating, disrespectful, and rampant. I love texting for a lot of reasons, but one shitty thing people often do is break up with someone by simply not texting them back. I'm sure it happened in other mediums in previous generations—it's an ageless dynamic that gets back to how it's healthy and helpful to be direct. If you've gone out with someone multiple times and don't want to keep seeing them, tell it to them straight. Simply assuming someone will get the message when you fail to return their texts is both unkind and contributes to the bad practice of hoping someone will read your mind so you don't have to speak it. On the other hand, it's totally okay to go radio silent on people you have a good reason to cut off. People often use texts as a form of harassment—if someone is making you feel unsafe or bad about yourself, by all means, deploy the radio silence. You don't owe an explanation to anyone who's trying to intimidate you.

16. Clean your sheets. Seriously.

Last Thoughts

In her work, writer bell hooks lays down an important starting point for healthy relationships: before you can have an equitable, honest, supportive relationship with someone else, you've got to learn to love yourself. That sounds simple, but it's tough. In fact, it's a pretty rare ability to feel a core confidence in who you are. That's thanks, in part, to the mixed messages we get from our culture. We're taught from a young age to "just be yourself," of course, but we're also constantly told what a perfect person looks like. Just be yourself, but make sure your true self is a long checklist of very specific things: loving, but not clingy; confident, but not selfish; beautiful, but not vain, or sexy. We're taught that we're supposed to believe in ourselves and that we'll never be good enough. Building healthy relationships with others means learning to ignore a lot of those nasty messages about how we're supposed to be.

We tell ourselves that being with anyone is better than winding up alone. For many people, that's just not the case. Even though many people do aim to be in a long-term relationship at some point, we shouldn't treat being single as a tragic limbo but as a time to appreciate independence and date different folks. I'm being very mature about all of this, of course, but I'm as prone to crying while watching bad TV alone as the next girl. Value being single as the opportunity it provides for reflection, exploration, and establishing good relationship habits. Practice being honest and commit to being direct. Then watch another episode of *Twin Peaks* and drink some whiskey. All of these things are possible.

MICHELLE TEA

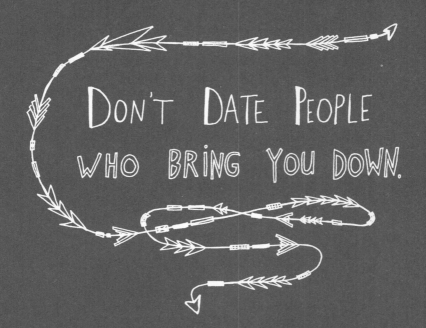

Don't Date People
who Bring You Down.

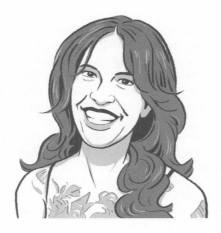

Michelle Tea is smaller than I thought she would be—she seems so big on the pages of her feisty fiction, like Rent Girl and The Chelsea Whistle. *We meet up for the first time in her natural habitat: a warm, dimly lit coffeeshop where she's about to take over the small stage to read from her book,* Valencia. *Michelle's prose draws from her own experiences, growing up queer in Boston in the '80s and hanging out with a love-hate crowd of punks, poets, and troublemakers in San Francisco. She recommends knowing your limits, making out with cute people, and learning life skills from ex-alcoholics.*

Don't Overthink Things.

You just know what you want, don't you? It's just about deciding to do something and doing it, not overthinking it.

I've definitely spent a lot of time in relationships that didn't feel good. I over-intellectualized them and came up with all sorts of reasons why I needed to stick with it: either that I was crazy or that it didn't matter that I didn't feel good. Now I would never do that. If it doesn't feel good, I get out of it.

I really know if I like somebody or not. Paying attention to how I feel is important because I can rationalize all kinds of things, but at the end of the day, it's a quality of life issue. Am I happier because of this person? Am I more stressed out because of this person?

At some point, I just thought, "Oh, relationships just make me anxious and people just stress me out and I'll always feel that in a relationship." I feel like I know now if I'm hanging out with someone who brings me a lot of happiness, versus if I'm hanging out with someone who brings me a lot of strife.

I recently decided to get pregnant. Having kids is something I've always felt really ambivalent about, so I needed to come to a resting place about how I felt about it. I thought, "If I had a partner, it's definitely something I would do." You can overthink having a kid more than you can overthink most things. There are lots of reasons to not have a kid; you can think a lot about those. But there are lots of great reasons to have kids, and I knew it was an experience I wanted to have. You just decide you're going to do it and you do it.

Getting pregnant is kind of a big scary thing to do by yourself, both financially and spiritually. But holding out and waiting for someone to have a baby with, when you're 40...you actually don't have the time for that. So I didn't discuss it with anyone, I wanted to make the decision on my own. The only person I talked about it with was my sister a little bit, since she has a three-year-old daughter. She was really supportive, which was really encouraging because she knows me better than anyone.

Some People Are Great for Make Outs, That's All.

Basically, it's just about what you want. What I was ultimately looking for when I was dating was sort-of-true love. I had this sort of ideal that I wanted, but I have this chronic openness to people. I like people, I'm curious about people, I find people adorable. So I was having to sort through all the people I was meeting—not everyone is marriage material. I had to come up with these sorts of categories for people. There are people who are good for sleeping with, there are people who are good to casually date, and there are people who are good to have relationships with. And those are totally different people and it's important not to confuse them.

I ultimately want a stable, monogamous relationship with someone I can build a world with. It's important that people I date long term are somewhat stable in themselves. For that kind of relationship, age is important; they have to live in the same town as me.

For casual dating, the person doesn't have to live in the same town as me, our ages can be a bit different, they don't have to be totally pulled together.

Someone I sleep with, they basically just have to be hot.

It's good for me to go into these interactions when I'm getting to know someone. Like, "Oh, this person's cute. There's something about them that seems super young. They don't live in the same town as me. So maybe we should just have a little affair and that will be that." Or, like, "This person seems really interesting, they kinda have their shit together, I'm going to date them and then see if they have the kind of character I'm looking for to build something more lasting."

As it's happens, things organically take their own shape. They either work or they don't. I was dating someone and then it got to the point where it was clear that it wasn't going to go deeper, so I ended the relationship because it would have been unhealthy to stay in it. I had a fling that was just a fun sex thing but then I started seeing someone I really cared about, so I ended that.

Sometimes you wind up falling for someone, but I have to ask myself, is this a safe person for me to fall for? If warning signs pop up, I'm going to end it—because I'm not interested in casually dating for 40 years.

Definitely Have Deal Breakers—And Stick to Them.
Not everything can be accommodated, nor should it need to be. My relationship history involves accommodating a lot of bullshit and it's taken me a long time to figure out that it's okay to have boundaries and get out of relationships that don't feel good.

Deal breakers for me: I'm less and less attracted to people who have these issues like untreated depression or an active alcohol or drug addiction. It's fine if people have depression or addictions and are actually dealing with it, but otherwise I have found that those people don't make good partners. Other deal breakers: Any time I feel bad around someone, it's a deal breaker. If someone has a mean streak, it's a deal breaker. If I have a boundary and they cross it, that's a deal breaker. If someone doesn't support my sobriety, that's a deal breaker. A deal breaker should be a big deal.

I had this dumb thing with this person I was dating this year where I had a boundary. I felt really proud of myself, I had a boundary where I said, "I don't want you to talk to me about your ex-girlfriend and how much of a jerk she was." That seems like an okay thing to ask of someone you're dating, but she just thought that was unreasonable, that she should be able to talk about her ex-girlfriend all of the time. So I let my boundary lapse. That's my pattern in relationships: To have a boundary, have it challenged, go "Okay, fine," then having a meltdown. And so I could see this coming: My boundary was challenged, I was going to have a meltdown and I thought, "This is stupid. I should just break up with them instead." So I did. And I was at peace.

Don't Date People Who Bring You Down—Even if They're Cute and Deep.

I'm attracted to people with emotional depth and for a long time, I mistook depression for emotional depth. But now I can recognize that and I'm actually repelled, though not in a judgmental way.

What feels healthy is someone who's dealt with their own shit. Whatever that is. Whatever crappy childhood or traumatic twenties is in their background that's made it hard for them, they've figured it out. They're a person who really likes life, not someone who's looking for another person to make them happy. And I'm looking for someone who's into me. Who's not threatened or critical, but is just like, "Oh my god, you're rad!" Someone who is open to being loved. A lot of people can't handle it, they can't handle vulnerability—they find it terrifying.

What feels healthy to me is someone who knows how to communicate, who doesn't get triggered or defensive. If I'm with someone who gets defensive, I'll respond in-kind and get really defensive. I've been in a lot of relationships where my focus has been, "Okay, don't get triggered just because they're triggered." When my focus maybe should have been, "Don't date someone who gets fuckin' triggered all the time!"

You can't go into dating someone all suspicious, all negative, but at the same time, understand that people are on their best behavior and you don't wholly understand who someone is if you've only known them for a little bit. If you're a fast mover, like I am, that's important. I tend to get to know people suddenly and powerfully. And that's nice, but you can't make plans based on that.

Figure Out Your Bad Patterns.
It's really easy to look back at your old relationships and say, "That person sucked." But it's really important to ask, "What was my part in it?" Maybe your part was just that you stayed in it. But that's important to know—I have the tendency to stay in shitty relationships. So how do I know a relationship is shitty? Because I feel anxious; I feel bad.

Most people grew up in crazy homes and as a result don't know how to be in a healthy relationship. And I've found AL-ANON, a group for friends and families of alcoholics, which is totally amazing. It's been my number one helper for figuring out how to make the relationship that I want. It helps you figure out what your needs are. It's taught me how to stand up for my needs, how to have boundaries, how to walk away from things that don't work. It's a lot of people just trying to figure out how to deal with people problems.

I've done a lot of making lists about what I'm looking for, writing about what went wrong in a relationship and what I did. That's really important.

What are my patterns? What sort of negative things do I bring into a relationship? What sort of things do I do to sabotage my own happiness? What's common about the people I date? It's about really looking at yourself honestly. If I'm dating and not looking at my tendencies, I'm going to keep bringing in people who keep repeating those patterns. But when you're able to see your own behavior more clearly, you just don't allow it to happen again and again and realize that you bring part of the equation.

TRACY CLARK-FLORY

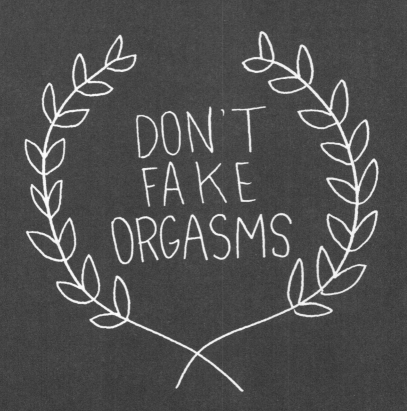

DON'T
FAKE
ORGASMS

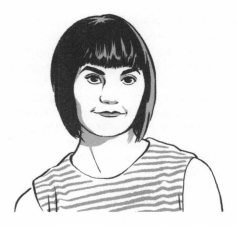

The San Francisco Ferry Building is so swirling with people that Tracy Clark-Flory and I can't even find a place to sit. We eventually perch on a bench outside Peet's Coffee, a throng of commuters, tourists, and screaming babies surrounding our small, intimate conversation. No one notices us amid the chaos. But if the tables nearby were eavesdropping, they'd likely be a little scandalized. Clark-Flory is the always-articulate Salon.com sex and gender staff writer—she digs into tricky subjects like hook-ups, rape culture, and sexting in a way that feels sincere and level-headed. I've always found her writing to be a refreshing counter-point to moralizing on sex and dating and am excited for the chance to buy her a cup of coffee. Over the San Francisco morning chaos, we talk about pleasure, myths, and a deal with the devil.

Don't Fake Orgasms.

I wish I could hit my twenty-year-old self over the head. Come on. Don't fake orgasms.

When I was 24, I wrote an essay for Salon called, "In Defense of Casual Sex," really in defense of exploration. That whole phase in my life was about testing out different people, seeing how I felt about them and seeing how they reacted to me in the real adult world. The experiment was really positive in that sense. Most of the guys I dated were not really great relationship material, but I really liked most of them. I got great, enriching experiences from even very casual relationships.

But the major thing I learned was the peril of prizing my partner's pleasure over my own. It's so unfulfilling and such a charade. What a waste of time. I never, ever want to do that again.

Dating was a total performative act; I was totally concerned about wanting to be desired. So much of my sexual identity was about feeling like I had some sort of sexual power. There was a lot of faking it, not just sexually but, like, trying to be the person that I thought they would like—being cool and confident, not too clingy. I think that approach made sense in that context because none of them was really looking for a relationship, and neither was I; so both of us wearing our armor was a kind of self preservation.

My most recent relationship is when all of that stuff fell away. I'm not afraid to be myself, to be dorky, neurotic, a little crazy, and have no worries about whether he likes me or not. Part of it is being with someone who's totally available to be in a relationship, there's no worry that I'll scare him off. It's so nice to not be in that place of turning text message interactions over and over with your friends. God, what a waste of time.

If He Runs Away, Let Him Run.

When I was in that early twenties phase, I was attracted to people who were totally unavailable—they were dating other people, they were running away from intimacy, they were guys who were similarly layering on the armor to protect their ego. That was in part because people who are available are kind of terrifying. Intimacy is actually pretty scary!

When you're chasing someone who's running away, there's no chance of being challenged, there isn't a mutual interaction where both people are made vulnerable. When you're chasing someone who's unavailable, there's rejection, but the degree of rejection from someone who you're actually in a relationship with, who actually knows you, it's so much higher. Once you're in a relationship and let someone fully know you, they can actually fully reject you. And that's what's terrifying.

I realized how scary it can be to date someone who's totally available and wants to be with you, but I've also come to realize how wonderful that can be once you move past the fear. Do the work of saying the things that need to be said, expressing yourself, and allowing yourself to be normal.

Now I think: Don't chase after anyone; You shouldn't have to. Romantic movies all revolve around the premise of running after someone, but I don't think that's actually a very good idea.

Unravel Your "Ideal Partner" Myth.
Right now I'm working on challenging my idea of an ideal partner. The type of partner I've always seen myself ending up with has been this person who has all the parts of my personality: He would be an intellectual, who was also sensitive, also an artist, career-minded but also emotionally intelligent, caring, and supportive. Now I'm thinking, okay, what are the most essential parts? What can I actually not live without? What traits do I really need long term?

I've never fantasized about a wedding, ever, but I realized recently that I've had this ideal partner in my head for much of my life. So even without buying into the whole marriage thing, there still are these myths I've created and live with. Right now I'm in a place of trying to figure out what parts of this story I've told myself are things I want to hold onto.

I desperately want to know what qualities I must find in a partner to have a long-term, satisfying relationship. Everyone claims to have the answers, but I'm not sure there is any one right set of answers, so it's been a lot of self-scrutiny.

I've had lawyer boyfriends who present an enormous intellectual challenge, and there is something really energizing about that. But then, my job is intellectually challenging. So at the end of the day, do I want to come home to some intellectual combat? Or do I want to come home to someone I can connect with on a more emotional, caring level? I don't know what I'll find ultimately, whether I need that or don't.

It's so cliché and I hate to play into this, but post-25 I suddenly started feeling like, "I don't have time to fool around anymore, I want to settle down." I hate it! But it's how I feel! That's so conventional! And I'm not conventional in a lot of ways, but I've realized that it's important to me to become a mom. It's there, it's true! Honestly, this year, my dial on that got cranked up. I start to panic about how much money I'm making, whether I'll be able to make enough money to actually support a family. It's become a big part of my current relationship, thinking: Will he be able to be an equal partner in owning a home and raising a kid?

I feel like I've shifted profoundly since just a few years ago. Casual sex and dating is now just so unappealing, I have no interest in going out to bars and meeting people. A year and a half ago, I was not even looking for a boyfriend, and now I'm like: "Children!" It's crazy!

I do wonder if there's some biological element to it, something chemical or hormonal. I have friends who, when we talk about marriage and kids, they're like, "Ugh, no." But I feel really strongly about what I want. I'm fully aware that I don't want to be a mom right now, but I know that's what I want at some point.

Talk About Sex.

One partner I had, on paper he seemed like: "This is the man you should marry." He was so emotionally intelligent, very sweet and sensitive, also had a writing career, was family-minded. But sexually, we were such a mismatch. I was questioning myself for feeling that way, telling myself like, "God, can't you just get over this one thing?" We came to the conclusion that we were so different that we just couldn't work it out.

We had a desire issue; he wanted sex much less than I did. But the real thing was that he was so uncomfortable talking about sex. And I'm like, I write about sex. It's so important to me to be able to talk openly about sex. For him, it was almost like there was a block. He could talk about it intellectually, we could talk hypothetically about sex in culture and have really challenging conversations, but we couldn't talk about our own lives.

It's important to be on the same page with sex. I feel like the guy I'm with now...we're a perfect sexual matchup. The attitude he has toward sex and the way he thinks about it, he doesn't feel weighed down with guilt or shame. It feels like we're speaking the same language, there isn't that extreme effort of translation. Just: You get it, I get it, we're on the same page.

My mom has officially told me that she hates it when I describe her as a hippie, so they're, um, Berkeley liberals. My parents were always open about expressing that being sexually compatible was one of the most important and sustaining parts about their relationship; that it's the glue of marriage. That was important information for me because I have so few friends whose parents are still together and my parents love each other and they're best friends.

Prince Charming Is A Scam.

My mom would always talk about how when a woman marries a rich man, it's a deal with the devil. It doesn't come for free. That kind of inequity in a relationship can bring up all sort of problems and I don't want to see the gender-flip of that happen to me—I need my partner to come to the table with an equal amount.

My mom's example was always my grandma, who lived a pretty isolated life. She was miserable. Her husband, my grandfather, was a successful businessman. They didn't really even like each other; they weren't real partners; they weren't real friends. She did not have the personal capital or ability to leave and be on her own. Her marriage was a business deal that left her miserable for her entire life. My mom would tell me this tragic story about when my grandma was on her deathbed, dying of cancer, and called the whole family into the room. She told everyone that basically she had been waiting for a second chance at life. She said, "I've been waiting for a better life, a second life." She had thought that my grandfather would die first and at least she would get some time to live her own life. That was an extreme cautionary tale for me growing up.

As a woman, you get all these messages that this prince in shining armor is going to show up and save you. Even now, there's this narrative of being saved by marriage. You'll get married and everything will be great and easy. But what an unfair expectation! One thing my parents instilled in me is that a partner should bring a whole lot to your life, but they shouldn't be your whole life. No one else can make you happy or can fix your life. You have to save yourself. It means a lot to me that I can pull my own weight and do my best.

2.

Building Feminist Relationships

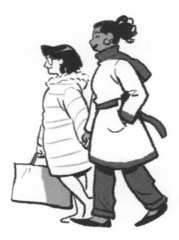

I have a life-long fear of becoming a bitter and unappreciated housewife.

I don't think I'm alone in this, but my friends do tell me sometimes that this fear is absurd. When they tell me I'm being ridiculous to worry about winding up trapped and sad in a relationship, I can only start ranting about the history of women in the world. I'll refrain from launching into this spiel, but it starts with shouting about graveyards where the women's tombstones bear only his name and the word "Mrs." Long story short, I don't think it's an irrational fear, and it's led to some hard-and-fast rules with boyfriends over the years.

Unless I'm feeling exceptionally generous, I won't wash my boyfriend's dishes. I won't do his laundry. I won't pay his rent. I won't let him go angry and silent for long—we've got to talk about feelings. I won't post kissy, cutesy photos of us online. There are a hundred concrete behaviors like this that are meant to ward off both becoming a doormat and becoming a woman whom others define by her boyfriend. I thought if I could put together a strong enough collection of specific feminist habits, I could build a relationship free of sexism. It turns out it's more complicated than that.

Every relationship I've been in has made me realize new ways that cultural expectations around gender affect both my behavior and my partner's. Just by refusing to do some dishes, I can't unwind the string of stories that society sews into us in a million ways.

Sometimes when my mind is stuck on something sad, I call up my aunt Paula, who grew up in the fifties and sixties and now lives on a tiny island off the coast of Maine. One winter I was in love with the guy I was dating—like full-body, no-eye-on-the-exit-door kind of love—and he broke up with me. Part of his problem was that I'm so extroverted, forward, and confident, and I have a busy life; he's more low-key and introverted. "You're so strong," he said. "You should date someone who appreciates that."

I called up Paula. I told her I was upset by that voice in my brain that says my relationships would be better if I could just figure out how to make the guy happy. As much as I try to act the way I want to act, I'm haunted by the persistent mental version of that ubiquitous *Cosmo* headline, an irritating refrain that constantly prods, "Transform your love life by learning these 75 ways to please your man."

"That's depressing," Paula said. "Is dating really like that? I thought my generation made it so you wouldn't feel that way."

Sadly, yes, these bad ideas are still the way my brain thinks sometimes. It's not fair, but it's real. Her generation's work and activism has given people my age the tools to recognize that the pressure to build relationships around what men want is a sexist expectation—and that those imbalanced power dynamics don't help anyone. We now have the language to talk about sexism in relationships, we have better role models for what expectations are healthy, and we have the support to strive for more equitable relationships without feeling crazy and alone. But the problems my parents' generation dealt with still permeate our love lives. Sexism is both gigantic and subtle. This is work that never ends. Dang it.

In my mid-twenties, I began a great long-term relationship with Carl. Now, he is arguably one of the most supportive boyfriends on the face of the Earth. But it still took about two years into our relationship for me to speak up about the things I didn't like. How did it take years of dating to tell him that I felt disrespected by the way he would tell me how to cut onions properly? Or that his harsh tone of voice during our conversations sometimes made me sad? Why didn't I feel the ability to just speak up? That tendency to bite my tongue when I don't have anything nice to say is a deeply engrained bad habit. Part of it comes from me being immature and chicken, sure, but a lot of that hesitancy to take up my boyfriend's time and space stems from the intense cultural teaching that I should take care of my partner's needs rather than articulate my own. I should be happy with what I can get and if I don't have anything nice to say, I shouldn't say anything at all.

To his immense credit, whenever I did speak up about my needs and desires, Carl took them seriously and thought deeply about how his own behavior impacted me. We worked out some guidelines that were bigger than my no-dishes-and-laundry rules: Carl needed to be more respectful and I needed to complain more.

That old head-over-heels boyfriend was right: I do need to only date people who appreciate how strong I am. And when we're together, I need to be even stronger.

The Details

Conversations around dating as a feminist often turn to questions about whether it's okay to dress sexy and who should pick up the check at dinner. Those are both things to think over, sure, but they're the tip of the iceberg. They're the tippy-top bits of the hulking mass of expectations we have around the way people are supposed to act.

Feminism isn't just about gender and it's certainly not just about what clothes you should wear. I use feminism as the name for the process of recognizing the social rules of our society, discussing where they come from, and deciding which to break. In addition to gender, we have a lot of rules that guide our assumptions around race, class, sexuality, ability, and physical appearance (just to name a few).

People of my generation have a tendency, I've found, to walk around feeling like a "bad feminist" because we don't always do things in a way we think is "feminist." I have friends who feel bad about dressing sexy and friends who feel bad about not wanting to dress sexy. I have many friends who are uncertain about how to respectfully flirt with people. I feel this worry a lot, too; like if I diverted the amount of brain energy that I spend worrying about whether the guy I have a crush on will text me back to worrying about social justice, I could create world peace, and therefore I am wasting my life and am a terrible feminist. But composing a list of things that are 100 percent feminist and things that are 100 percent unfeminist will drive you crazy and result in a bunch of useless rules. It's more helpful to examine *why* we want what we want. It's useful to examine what perspectives our desires and actions take into account—and what perspectives we leave out.

Relationships are about both those daily decisions we make in our heads—whether to tell your boyfriend you're angry or whether to sleep with someone after one date—and the slow, giant life decisions we make over time—like whether to have kids or whether to break up with your girlfriend. Its focus is on the big social and economic pressures that guide these decisions. They're hard to see, lurking under the water, but they explain why we often run aground.

Twenty Lessons to Learn from People in Feminist Relationships

1. **Feminism isn't just for women.**

   This is obvious, but let's start here. Sexism affects *all* of us negatively in relationships. We're all told not to talk about feelings, especially guys. Being honest is so damn hard. The consequences about being honest about how we feel are steep: being vulnerable exposes us. Women often do the emotional work of encouraging men to open up and talk about their feelings because it's hammered into men that not expressing emotion is the masculine thing to do. But clamming up isn't doing anyone any favors.

2. **Be up front about your politics.**

   Iowan Rachel brings up that she works at a rape and domestic violence hotline, which some guys found weird and unsettling. Her boyfriend Martin was supportive and understood why her work was important. "It's nice to know there are men out there who are comfortable talking about those things, not just nodding but actually replying to you. I need someone who's going to support me in those things, not take it as an assault on all men everywhere that I'm deeply troubled by rape culture."

3. **Think about privilege.**

   I have a lifetime ban on dating white dudes who think they got where they are just by working hard. Personally, I would recommend this ban. It once kept me from sleeping with a guy who flirted by reading me passages of *The Fountainhead*. That's a silly example but, really, there's a lot here. So much of our culture is built around the myth that all people are able to pull themselves up by their bootstraps to radically transform their lives all on their own. That idea leaves so much off the radar— building precisely the life you want is just easier if you grew up white, male able-bodied, and with money. Think about the ways in which you feel comfortable that other people might not feel comfortable because of the assumptions heaped upon them when they were born. Recognize the parts of yourself that you feel ashamed about and the things your partners might be grappling with and just think about why those are issues.

4. **Recognize the power dynamics behind being competitive.**

   Our media constantly instills in us this idea that women need to compete against each other to "snag" a man. There is, I swear, an entire genre of made-for-TV Christmas movies just about two women fighting over who gets to celebrate Christmas with the hot male lead. This perception is pervasive and destructive. Our culture tells us that some women are thieves and others are heartbreakers and others are sluts. Don't play that stupid game and, if you're male, don't buy into it. "To me, women are on a team. I hope that I'm on a team with everyone, but especially women," says queer Portlander Choya. "I understand why women get catty and compete and, for me, I think it has to do with separating ourselves from people who are penalized by sexism (women) and aligning ourselves with people in power (men). Divide and conquer makes women weaker." Recognize that there are dark and powerful forces working against women being friends with women and counteract that with an extra dose of honesty, support, and compassion.

5. **Flirting is a treasured pastime.**

   People of all genders have told me that they feel

awkward about flirting because it puts you out on the line. But being respected and being a good friend shouldn't be at odds with being sexy. There's places where it's troublesome to express sexual interest in people—like, for example, your office—but outside of that, appreciate how flirting with someone can create a good sort of sexy energy. If flirting with someone is not fun and exciting, but instead driving you crazy and leading to a rollercoaster of emotion, that's a red flag. But otherwise, flirting can be a safe and positive way to express your sexuality.

6. **STFU.**

Several people had told Portland tech entrepreneur Matthew that he took up a lot of space in conversations, with friends, and also with his girlfriend. He developed a four-letter method for being a better human after reading the work of bell hooks: STFU. The letters stand for "Share time" (instead of dominating a conversation, recognize that you can be silent and listen), "Three seconds" (give people three seconds to chime in on a discussion before you jump in), "Find empathy" (really listen to people and think about where they're coming from) and "Understanding is not necessary" (meaning, you don't have to fully understand why someone feels a certain way, just take them at their word and spend some time thinking about it). He says it has helped him a lot to give friends and partners more space in conversations to air their feelings and ideas.

7. **Call yourself whatever you want.**

More and more, people get caught up on what to call themselves and their partners. Is she your girlfriend? Is he your friend? The problem is we don't have a large enough vocabulary to sum up the variety of relationships people build for themselves. People use a variety of cobbled together terms to describe the relationships that don't fall into "non-sexual, platonic friend" and "long-term boyfriend or girlfriend." Some that I've heard are "sex friend," "friend I sleep with," "partner," "my person," "date," "lover," "sweetie," "person I'm dating" and (one of my favorites), "the HELP (Homosexual Essential Life Partner)." One summer I had a "partner in crime" and that description worked pretty well. Rather than feeling pressure to squeeze your relationship into whatever definitions are well known, recognize that lots of people have great relationships that fall somewhere in that hard-to-describe zone—having sex with a friend who never becomes your "boyfriend" is a perfectly valid relationship that can be fun and positive as it is.

8. **Talk about what being a partner means.**

So you get to make up whatever labels you want, but the people involved need to be on the same page about what the relationship means. If you decide you want your relationship to change with a date/partner/sweetie/friend, talk about what the relationship means to you. If you're "just friends," does that mean you don't have sex? If you're "dating" does that mean you're monogamous? If you're "partners" does that mean you plan to meet each other's families? For some people, being a "girlfriend" means you plan to move in together some day—for other people that's not what they want to consider at all. Get concrete about your boundaries and expectations about time commitment, sex, personal space, and family rather than assuming the other person will have the same definition of your relationship.

9. **Protect your identity.**

My mom has this great story about spending hours one summer watching her boyfriend drive his motorcycle up and down the street. He was excited about motorcycles and it took her a while to realize that she was bored by trying to participate in that part of his life. There's a tendency to have our interests consumed by our partners' and to modify our behavior to match theirs. It's a tricky balance to support your partners' passions while becoming involved in the parts of their life that we genuinely want to without being subsumed by them.

10. **Speak up.**

Almost everyone has trouble telling their partners when they're doing something we don't like, but perceptions of complaining have a definite gender bias. There are a lot of negative words specifically describing women who speak up—nag, shrew, bitch—while men who speak out about what they want tend to be seen as assertive, confident leaders. Whatever your gender, push yourself to speak up when there's a problem in the relationship that's grating on you. Don't suffer in silence, hoping that a destructive habit or disrespectful behavior will change.

11. **You should be on the same team.**

There will *always* be points of conflict to speak up about. We carry so much shame and ridiculous baggage around with us. To get to the roots of why we do what we do, we've got to be up for talking about stuff we feel bad about without worrying that the other person is going to cut and run. "Being in a relationship means, 'Let's talk about it,'" says queer Portlander Choya. "We're on the same team. When he told me he cheated on me, I said, 'What are *we* going to do about it?" If anyone in the relationship is having a problem, you've got to talk about it and not feel ashamed.

12. **Embrace conflict.**

Ugh, I realize this sounds like something an annoying yoga teacher would say. But it's another way to think about needing to speak up about issues. My natural tendency is to try and steer as far clear of conflict as possible—and that just leads to me changing my behavior to cope with a partner, rather than addressing an issue head-on and asking them to make a change. People older and smarter than myself say that leads to resentment and they're right. They encourage me to see conflict as inevitable and natural. Use those as a chance to talk about differences between you and the ways you approach the world.

13. **Give each other space to talk about problems.**

Hand-in-hand with this idea of speaking up about problems is making sure everyone in the relationship is speaking up and feels listened to. Many people run into the issue of starting serious conversations in the middle of the night, when one person is too tired to focus, or in the middle of a discussion about some logistical issue (a conversation about what to get at the store turns into a big discussion over "the principle of the thing," for example). There's never a "good" time to talk about difficult stuff, but it's always ideal to choose a time when all involved have the ability to focus. Many people say their relationships are helped by intentionally making time to talk about the things they're afraid to talk about, so that one person doesn't wind up having their concerns shut down or dismissed by another.

14. **Sex isn't perfect.**

I've talked with a lot of women who faked orgasms for years in relationships with men. These were loving, fulfilling relationships in many ways, but the women just weren't getting off and either didn't feel comfortable speaking up about what they wanted or just weren't sexually attracted to their partners enough to orgasm even when they could talk openly. And I've talked with numerous guys who were crushed to find out that their girlfriends had been faking orgasms, sometimes just occasionally and sometimes for years. Faking an orgasm is a sign that something is not right—that someone doesn't feel safe enough in the relationship to be honest, that there's undue pressure to have sex that ends in orgasms, that someone has some stigma attached to talking about what they want sexually, or that your sexual needs are just incompatible. Don't go there in a long-term relationship. It never ends well. If you are faking them, recognize that it's a sign and think about what's motivating your need to pretend the sex is perfect.

15. **Be the partner you want to be.**

We have some pretty bunk cultural ideas about what a "perfect girlfriend" and "perfect boyfriend" should be like. It can be hard not to just accept our partners' ideas about what a relationship should look like and use them as our own. Learning healthy traits from our partners is great, of course. But there's a tendency to be drawn into the orbit of the people we love and acting more the way we think they want us to act. Learning the good habits while avoiding the holding pattern of becoming another person's image is lifelong work.

16. **Wear whatever you want, date whomever you want.**

Wear the boots, wear the skirt, wear leggings for pants and date your next-door neighbor. Just be intentional about it and be aware of when you're playing into old school ideas about the ways that women and men should be. When you're dressing and dating in a way that lines up with your beliefs, more power to you.

17. Money makes everything stressful.

In the United States in the late 1800s, single women moved away from home for the first time and got jobs in big cities and started earning paychecks that just barely covered rent. Young women were so poorly paid that if they wanted to go out for food and drinks, they had to rely on men to pick up the tab. The economic trend continues today, with women earning far less than men. Many women in long-term relationships with men they don't love explain the reason that they're still in the relationship is simple: economics. Men can be good providers; they can provide support. But whether it's women relying on men to pay the rent or men leaning on women, economic inequity leads to unequal relationships and that creates tension.

18. See the invisible jobs.

All this big picture talk about respecting each other and speaking up can get eclipsed by mundane tasks. How you take up space and think about how to run your lives can boil down to the tiny level of who thinks to wash the dishes and who thinks ahead enough to buy toilet paper. For all their good, feminist discussions and intentions, many people say, relationships run aground on these infuriating daily issues. Many people resolve these kinds of debates—over who makes dinner and who cleans—with concrete and regular discussions of what needs to get done and how each partner needs to pull their own weight. Lots of couples divide up chores between each other based on what they like to do. Many times, though, women in straight relationships wind up taking on more than an equal share of domestic tasks, including more time spent on childcare and cleaning the house. This isn't necessarily a problem, if the person doing the extra works likes the chores and feels like their partner picks up the slack in some other way, but energy spent to take care of a house and family is often invisible because there's no paycheck attached and it's not appreciated as actual work.

19. Children raise the stakes.

All these issues about personal space, desires, housework, and discussing conflict become much more compressed when you have kids. Many people who've had 'em have less time to sit and talk about issues with their partner. There's suddenly a lot more house and domestic work to be done as you wash mountains of diapers and have to feed an extra mouth. Money often becomes increasingly tight, and there are a million important decisions to make every day while raising a child. Being pregnant and having kids in many ways makes women more economically vulnerable. Raising a child and going through pregnancy is so expensive that many women say they stay in unhealthy relationships longer because they need someone to pitch in to help raise the child or pay the bills. People with kids work out their own ways to talk about big-picture relationship issues. Some couples carve time out of the week to have a family discussion or just personal, alone time. Setting a sacred time of the week to be alone can be a good idea, as is having a standing time once a week to talk about the conflicts and issues, large and small, that develop.

20. **Sexism is big, subtle, and real.**

So are: racism and homophobia and body shame— these assumptions creep into our behaviors and wield a control in our heads that's hard to see. All the advice here is about recognizing and dealing with the impacts of those destructive ideas, and how we should think about people and ourselves. It's hard to parse out exactly why we act the way we do. Why is it hard for some people to open up about their feelings? Why do some people always feel bad about sleeping with someone new? Why do we spend so much mental energy worrying about exes, but work to understand that the power structures of our society reverberate all the way down to the micro relationship level? What feels small, special, and wholly our own is still affected by those outside biases in ways that are hard to pinpoint and even harder to root out.

Last Thoughts

When we talk about feminist approaches to dating, we can get really hung up on terms. I find that people—myself included—go around feeling like we're "bad" feminists because of what we want in relationships. But for me, it doesn't matter what you call yourself. It matters how you're living in the world. I describe my own feminism as a process of recognizing the rules of society, articulating them, figuring out which ones I should break, and then deciding how to break them. That means talking about everything from the ways that movies are more likely to give screen time to white dudes than anybody else, to the ways that I privilege male opinions over my own ideas in my own relationships. A lot of the ways that our society functions is pretty screwed up, and a lot of the way things are unequal comes down to the rules about who is important and who's not. I think it's important to recognize that the daily actions involved in challenging these ideas are really tough. Feeling strong enough in yourself to speak up for what you want in your relationships—regardless of your gender—is something many people find to be difficult. I wish we could get to a point where we can plant a victory flag and declare success, but this is deeply personal work that never ends.

Sometimes, to me, all the big issues of sexism just feel like too much. I'm never going to fix all the inequality in the world—some days, all the ways gender is policed feels futile to challenge. How are my boyfriend and I ever going to have an equitable relationship with hundreds of years of patriarchy pushing against us? When I feel low like that, I return to this most basic place: getting comfortable with who I am. Some days, just figuring out how to love myself is radical enough. Other days, when I'm feeling good, I've got more fight in me. Regardless of where I'm at, helping people out with their own struggles makes me stronger myself. Talking through my relationships with friends I trust always buoys me. That's a big part of what I've learned: creating healthy, happy, feminist relationships is too big a weight to carry on your own. I've got to have a support system, a network of people who I can be honest with and who make me feel good about myself even when everything in the entire world is rotten. A lot of discussions about relationships focus on the individual. But we're not going to get very far by ourselves.

AYA dE LEON

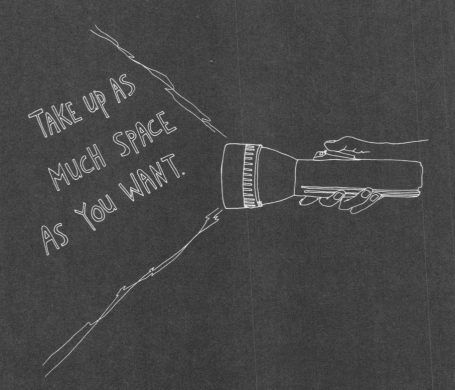

TAKE UP AS MUCH SPACE AS YOU WANT.

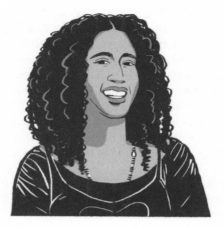

Aya de Leon is a long-time activist and poet who spent her twenties living in the San Francisco Bay Area, surrounded by performers, outspoken feminists, and queer folks. Now, a decade after her busiest time on stage, Aya has a husband, a young daughter, and a lot of thoughts about how to carve out the life she wants.

Being in a relationship with a male partner has taught her a lot about sexism and how it works at close range. However, as a feminist and a woman of color, it's also taught her to walk her talk when the issues in her relationship are complicated or unexpected. Aya is a Black and Latina woman born in America, while her partner is a Black and South Asian man who was born in the UK and raised in the Caribbean. "While the sexism in our relationship gets very thick at times, I have also learned to track the places where my own privilege in the relationship sits as the person from the U.S. with an immigrant partner," Aya told me, as we talked over the phone on a rainy winter day. "I always seem to have the home court advantage." She is careful to note that her criticisms of his behavior can easily read as a critique and dismissal of his culture—she has to find a place between speaking up about her feelings and watching out for an "I-know-better" assumption. Aya insists on having a big, powerful life despite the tangle of race, class, gender, and cultural issues that make it difficult to be herself and, at the same time, her partner demanding space for his unassimilated, unedited West Indian self. "Amidst the battles, we find ourselves trying to build a loving relationship and family across these differences. And we find ourselves succeeding. On good days, I love him more than I ever thought possible. On bad days, I wonder what the hell I've gotten myself into," says Aya.

Take Up As Much Space As You Want

My partner and I were together for about a year and change, then we moved in together, and then we almost killed each other. Then we worked through that, then we got married, and then we almost killed each other. Then we worked through that, then we had a kid, and then we almost killed each other again. And then we worked through that.

I have high standards for how I think men should treat women and how women should be able to be. That was the source of a lot of friction. I was unwilling to make my life any smaller.

I want to have integrity in my values as a feminist in my relationship, and what's required for this is shifting my values a little and my relationship a lot. I feel much more like we're peers in this process now. He's pushed himself to take on different challenges and it's been interesting seeing us figure out how to back each other more.

I think the one piece of advice I would definitely give myself in this relationship is that when you're feeling very much in love with this person, and there are things going on that you notice and don't like but, emotionally, you're feeling so lovey-dovey that you don't want to rock the boat, rock the boat anyway. You need to establish a better baseline of expectation. That might have saved me some difficultly.

It's Not Actually Humiliating To Go After What You Want

Twelve years ago, I was at the height of my public life as a spoken-word performing artist. I was 33 and I had made it onto this big slam team. For the male artists around me, success translated into a ton of romantic offers. But being a feminist badass, with an interest in dating men, did not translate into anything romantically for me. If anything, it was difficult to navigate. That was in part because of my own insecurities but also because most of my social interactions would be part of my public life.

A lot of time, I'm at these events and I'm performing. At one point in the event, I'm on stage and I'm killing it. At another point, I'm hanging around with people and I see someone who's interesting or attractive. The lights are dim. But then it's awkward not knowing that person and what their story is—are they single? Who are their friends? What's their sexual orientation? To talk to that person and get even three minutes of private conversation would seem really forward. When you have a public role in a scene, there's no sense of privacy.

I should have been a little bit more of a mac. There was some fear I had about being embarrassed, like I was worried I would hit on someone and they wouldn't be interested. I was definitely a bit timid and needed someone to show their interest first. Instead, I should have been thinking, "What am I interested in? What do I want?" and going boldly out there. It's not actually humiliating to go after what you want.

I started internet dating as a way of meeting people outside of the public part of my life. At the time, in 2001, it wasn't nearly as common as it is now. There was something useful about someone having to articulate something, like, "I am X and I am looking for X because X." You could at least have some declaration. In the world I was in there were a lot of cool people hanging out, but that it was unclear who was dating someone or what anybody wanted.

I posted an ad on Craigslist that my now-partner answered. It was the first time I was in love—no holds barred, no back door open. This was the time when I was like, "Bam!" He and I really grew up together in a lot of ways. It was the first time he had ever been in love *and* been present—earlier in his life he had been in love but had been drinking a lot. So this was the first time that he was able to feel what it feels like to be close to somebody.

When we moved in together, that was it for me. I'm moving in and I never want to move out, so that means I'm here, I'm committed. It was hard, but I was determined. I had the perspective that relationships are hard. He had the perspective: fuck this, it's too hard.

Honor Your Role In Your Family—Don't Drown In It
You know, the bottom line of all of this is we just both come from significant trauma histories. Anytime people come from significant trauma histories, relationships are hard. Getting into a relationship when I was older, having been alone for a lot of that time and focused on my own life, I had a lot of resistance set up to the sexism of a relationship with a man. But I was unprepared for how bad it would be at times. There are at least 100 major highlight moments of

the relationship where I could capture the moment with, "Really?"

My generation of women watched our moms get hit with sexism a lot of the time. There's some ways that I watched my mom and said, "Wow, that's really stupid. Why are they putting up with that? I would never put up with that." Now I'm able to see some of the structural things that were operating on our moms that made it difficult to resist effectively.

My mom had a partner for years who, especially around cleaning the house, had this attitude of, "I make a mess and somehow magically it gets cleaned up." I remember my mom being, like, "I'm not the maid!" I didn't learn how to team up with a partner to keep a house in working order, but I learned how you fight. You fight and scream and yell to keep from being taken advantage of in terms of domestic labor.

What's interesting is some forms of sexism are on the surface: you read the label of a guy when you get into the relationship. Other types develop slowly over time, as you get deeper into the relationship. Then it's harder to be like, "What is this? I'm getting out."

The kinds of labor that women do in heterosexual relationships are invisible, like holding together a community and organizing things for the family. So, like, a woman will be seen as "just chatting on the phone" but actually she's holding down the social life or the logistics of a family. I'm always the one whose tracking is on—how much food is there in the refrigerator? What do we need? And his just isn't.

Once you have a kid, it shifts everything and makes women so much more vulnerable. That's part of why I put it off so long, because my feminist training had taught me that you want to have as much political, economic, personal, and community network power as you can before you go into it. But even with all the resources I had amassed, it was astounding the way that having a kid increased the sexism in my relationship.

I knew that my kid would have a great mom—because I knew I would be a great mom—and that she would have one of the best black dads that I knew. Even if my partner decided to be a dick about our marriage, he has a big heart.

A key piece has been understanding that making a family go well takes work and leadership that I want to figure out how to honor—but not drown in.

We're like two bachelors living together, except that both of us are Oscar Madison and neither of us are Felix Unger.

There's an implicit sense coming from him that somehow I'm more responsible for things being neat, even though it's never quite articulated. It's never like, "Woman! Clean the house!" It's just like, "Wow, the house is so messy."

There's a subtlety around domestic work. It's not that he doesn't clean. He cleans sometimes. He cooks sometimes. But there's something there. Before we lived together, he kept his house neat. But once we moved in together, there were some expectations that once there was a woman involved, the cleaning fairies had been activated. After we became parents, the amount of mess increased ten-fold and the amount of time to deal with the mess decreased ten-fold.

The way we've worked through that is something that's surprised me: I've started to appreciate something about women's traditional work. Women who ran households and cooked had some skill there that my feminist mentors trained me to believe were not real skills. I'm in the process of figuring something out there, and figuring out what I want to ask from him, what skills do I need to learn, and taking charge of the management in order to provide an orderly and neat environment for my daughter. She's neither a Felix nor an Oscar, she's an innocent bystander.

I'm not saying I want to quit my job and be a full-time stay home mom, because I would go crazy. But if we decide that we should somehow be freed up from doing domestic work, either you've got to get the men to be doing that—and some of that is happening, though not as much as many women would like—or you're delegating it to immigrant women and poorer women and women of color. I have yet to pay anyone to clean my house and so there's this process of trying to figure out: what does justice look like? I'm still figuring that out.

Sexism Is Subtle

The biggest issue when we first moved in was his snoring. We moved into this apartment with this little built-in bed that became like an echo chamber. I told him, "Babe, you are snoring so loudly, it keeps me up. You need to address this." And he's like, "Eh, well, yeah." One of the things about sexism in intimate relationships is the sense of entitlement to women's resources. In this case, it was like, "Wow, you feel like you can just completely encroach on my sleep every night of the week and shouldn't have to be inconvenienced on any level to remedy that." There was no sense of, "I really care about you and I'm impacting you, so I'll take major steps to make sure that doesn't happen."

As is typical in those kinds of sexist situations, I figured out something I could do in the situation to fix it. I wore earplugs. But the snoring was so loud that the earplugs weren't enough. So I had earplugs, and then I had audio books with headphones that hooked over my ears. The sound of the audio book plus the earplugs drowned him out enough so that I could get to sleep.

That is so emblematic of sexism, but it's also so subtle. As sexism goes, it feels like it's not that big of a deal, but it's incredibly invasive and entitled.

When our daughter was a year old, he finally went to the doctor. They did a sleep study and the doctor was like, "Oh my God! We're surprised you're not dead. Your sleep apnea is so bad." Now he sleeps with a mask on and the sleep apnea is so much better. This was a serious situation. That's the thing about sexism—generally the things that women are asking for, from men, are not just good for the women but they're *also* good for the man. But male conditioning has made it so hard for men to do things like, for example, talk about their feelings or take responsibility for their health.

One good idea we've had is having a family meeting every Sunday morning. We started doing that because if you ask me what I think about something, I'll give you a treatise. If you ask him what he thinks about something, he'll give you a short answer, say, "I don't know, I have to think about it." On the one hand, I'm taking charge because he's ambivalent, slow, and not sure. But there also wasn't a lot of room for him. So the sexism would be how he would take the room—when he had a concern, he would feel like he deserved to air it right then. In parenting, there's not much time to discuss. So we decided to make a family meeting every Sunday that's like, this is the time to talk about finances, parenting, and values. It's a good system.

I think of my mentor, Puerto Rican feminist Aurora Levins-Morales. She taught me that we are in a particular period in history where women don't need to partner with men, but we can choose to. We can walk into relationships with men with our eyes open, knowing there will be sexism and disappointment and frustration, and we need and deserve a support system to help us through it. But we are also part of the historical moment of creating new possibilities between men and women. We have gotten to the point where we can imagine relationships with men that we can't quite make manifest yet. Our relationships are the frontlines, and we learn to arm ourselves with equal parts fierceness and love.

You Must Face The Avalanche ShitStorm Of Oppression

There were many days where I just felt like I was underneath an avalanche shitstorm of sexism and oppressive behavior. It's one thing to know sexism in the abstract and it's another thing to be in the middle of it.

The thing that has been powerful this year has to do with intersectionality. When I was a teenage feminist in the early eighties, I had a lot of second-wave feminism mentors. They were mostly white women who had a certain utopian fantasy version of marriage. Like, it should be that the man does 50 percent and he's a strong ally, and these are the only conditions under which marriage wouldn't be completely selling out. In some ways, the vision I was given was of a white, middle-class marriage where nobody has any trauma history or a lot of control issues, where no one yells and everyone talks in calm tones and is very reasonable. I can pretend to be that person and I have a lot of those skills, but I think men of color are much less assimilated into that middle-class communication style.

There was a place where I felt that I had to make a choice between my black family and an unrealistic set of ideals around sexism. I have compassion for my partner and myself about what it is we're trying to do, given the hurts that we've had and how hard it is to have a family when we're both children of divorce, abuse and neglect, and the way racism and genocide have made it hard to get close to people.

Even though the battle against sexism would write me a prescription of "fuck this, I'm out," there was something bigger that I wanted about having a black family and seeing sexism in a historical perspective. There was a piece around fighting racism in the fight to stay with my partner.

One thing I realized is that there was a lot of conflict in my marriage because I was not interested in manipulating my partner into making him feel like he's always in charge. I'm not interested in coddling his sense of entitlement. I was always challenging him and that's part of why we were always fighting.

ANDI ZEISLER

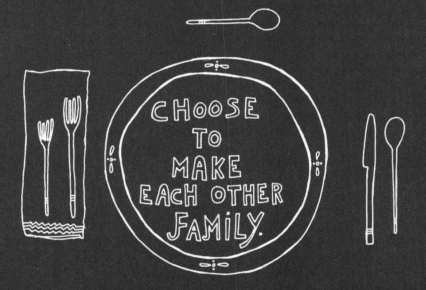

CHOOSE
TO
MAKE
EACH OTHER
FAMILY.

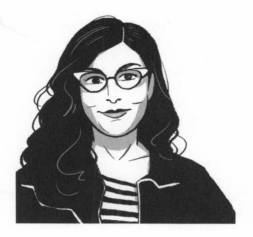

Andi Zeisler is ridiculously smart. She plays it cool, though. The co-founder of Bitch *magazine is one of those people who, as you're sitting together picking away at brunch omelettes, will talk off-the-cuff about her life and ideas in a way that's so eloquent that all you can contribute to the conversation is a couple "yeah"s and loud slurps of coffee.*

Andi founded Bitch *with friends when they were all in their twenties, living in the Bay Area and frustrated with the lack of discussion around pop culture representations of women, race, and class. These days, Andi is the author of two books, including* Feminism and Pop Culture, *is happily married, and has an adorable young son.*

Over breakfast at Portland's City State Diner, I munched on toast while she talked intelligently about marriage, independence, and the need to be impolite.

You Don't Have To Date A Ton Of People

The effort of dating, of meeting people, really wore me out. I'm a real introvert, I don't enjoy the feeling of needing to put myself out there. The whole thing of like, oh there's someone, I have to figure out whether they like me, I have to be in the same place as them, I have to look cute, I have to figure out things to talk about... I wanted it to just happen organically. But I felt like, "Dating is what I'm supposed to be doing, so I'm going to do it so I haven't left too many paths unexplored. I'm just going to say yes to people." I wasn't miserable, but it didn't feel like me and it never felt right. When I met my husband Jeffery, I told my mom, "I think this guy's really special." She was really dismissive, saying, "You're going to date hundreds of guys." I said, "That sounds terrible."

Jeffery and I have been married for ten years. I met him at a concert. I literally saw him across the crowded Greek Theater in Berkeley and was like, "I'm going to marry that guy with the tube socks and glasses." I was not in that mindset at all; it wasn't something I'd ever thought before. I just turned around and through a couple thousand people, saw him and thought, "There's something about that dude." Then I turned around and went about my business, I didn't even try to meet him.

I don't really believe in love at first sight. I'm superstitious and some things happen when they're supposed to happen. But I don't try to organize my life around the idea that fate happens.

At the theater, we bumped into one another and talked for two minutes, and then were like, "Okay, bye." What do you say in that situation? What am I going to do, ask him to come home with me? Then, when I left, I was in the BART station waiting to buy my ticket and he ran in and said, "Here's my number, I'm here for a few days. Call me."

I think we both felt an instant thing of, like, "I don't know you that well, but I know you're going to be important to me." It's an illustration of the idea that if you're not looking for love, that's what will happen.

In all of the relationships I'd had previous to that, there was a fundamental gut feeling that something was off. I was always ignoring my gut. This didn't have any of that, this felt really good right off.

Politeness Can Be Paralyzing

I was in a long-term relationship from when I was 23 till I was about 25. From the beginning, I didn't feel good about it. But I somehow felt compelled to stay in the relationship because I felt like, "This is what a relationship is supposed to be and I need to experience it." I wasn't punishing myself, I was just trying to make myself be what I thought was normal.

What I wanted to do at that time was sleep with a bunch of people and not have a boyfriend. But for some reason, I couldn't give myself permission to believe that was okay. So what I ended up doing was being in this relationship and just cheating on him a lot. It felt awful, but I felt like I'd committed to him at some point. After six months, I thought, "Well, I have to stick it out for at least a year."

We'd go down to Southern California to visit his family and his mother treated me like I was going to marry her son. She made me this soap cozy—this little knitted dress that goes over your soap, with "Andi's Kitchen" knitted on it. I was like, "Whoa, she really thinks this is happening." And then I realized, *he* thinks this is happening, too.

I think my default is to be polite and that gets me into a lot of goofy sitcom moments where I just can't get out of something. This was one of those moments. I was like, "Holy crap, this whole family thinks we're getting married and meanwhile I'm sleeping with someone else." Instead of being straight with him, I felt paralyzed. I did not want to admit to myself that maybe I am just not a person who wants a boyfriend. Maybe I just want to be alone and have guys to sleep with when I want to. I wasn't able to come to grips with the fact that that's what I wanted.

The first time he put his arm around me, we were walking down the street. It felt so wrong. I felt like my whole body was rejecting his arm, it was so heavy. And that was in the first four weeks of dating. So if I'd listened to myself, I would have said, "Let's just keep it casual" and gotten out of it. I look back and there were so many ways I could have mitigated that relationship if I'd had a better sense of myself or the language I wanted to use, or a feeling that I was entitled to something beyond that. The whole relationship became this snowball of bad choices, mostly on my part.

Be On The Same Page With Gender Roles

I used to work at Pottery Barn. It was such a bastion of heteronormativity, we called it Pregnancy Barn. Someone was always getting pregnant or getting engaged. I was privy to a lot of conversations about, like, how acceptable is a half-carat diamond? What's a proper proposal protocol? I felt like a real outlier, thinking those conversations were ridiculous.

Someone from Pregnancy Barn introduced me to this guy who lived in a fancy part of town, had a fancy job, and a fancy family. We dated for a little while, but I felt like I was being auditioned as a potential mate. At Pottery Barn, everyone was on the same trajectory: You go to college, you go to work, you get married, you ideally stop working. He was on that track and I was clearly not on that track.

There was something attractive about dating someone who had a good job, where going out to dinner wasn't like, "We need to split this burrito down the middle." But on the other hand, in that relationship I never felt comfortable.

My parents are of an older generation that is very gendered. When my father would spill something, he'd say, "Oh, honey, can you get a sponge and get that?" My mom was a real career lady—an executive at Revlon—and then when she and my dad got married, he was like, "No wife of mine is going to work" and she gave it up. I always grew up thinking, "Why should you have to do something just because he says to?"

Marriage Is As Feminist As Knitting

Jeffery asked me to marry him just about a year after we started dating. It wasn't on my mind. I thought we were going to have the kind of relationship where we dated forever and then finally got married because we wanted real plates, you know? I didn't grow up thinking marriage was the be-all end-all, and part of that's because my mother got married very late; she had me when she was 40. So his proposal totally surprised me. But it was not impulsive at all. He had really thought about it, he had a ring made and clearly waited a while. I was like, um, there's no discernible reason to say no and I can say yes and not have to have everything figured out. So, okay, let's do this.

And then, when I thought about marriage, it appealed to me in a way I never thought it would. We're choosing to make each other family.

The way I feel about marriage and feminism now is the way I feel about knitting. I like knitting and I'm a feminist who knits. But I would never say knitting is a feminist act. And I'm a feminist who's married, but I would never say getting married is a feminist act. It's hard to say, "I am going to bend this institution to fit my idea of feminism." You almost can't divorce marriage from its historical ideas about property and patriarchy. Those are built into it. I'm a feminist, my husband is a feminist, but saying that we have somehow made marriage feminist, I think that would be arrogant and presumptuous. You can't transform an institution that huge, and that has so much historical baggage. You can do things within a marriage to make it more egalitarian and feminist but it does not make marriage as an institution, feminist.

Make Space For Yourself

Everyone's marriage, unless you're Kim Kardashian, is private. You can't see from the outside what's going on within. We're independent people and big introverts, so in some ways, it's a very separate marriage. I've always said that my ideal living situation would be two little houses that are connected. We could live separately and choose whether or not to sleep in the same bed at night.

Jeffery and I don't spend that much time together. We probably spend like 45 minutes a day together. He works editing and retouching photos late into the night. Often he'll just fall asleep on the couch with the dogs or in the guest room. I think what's good is the sense of neither of us feels like, "You're my husband, you're my wife, therefore we must spend x amount of time together."

Since having a child, it's important for us to have family time. We spend a lot of time together on the weekends. We'll sleep in, eat breakfast, do some activity like go to the museum or the river where the kid can just run around. Then in the afternoon, we'll have family quiet time, where our son has to stay in his room for some time. That was a very conscious thing, because we needed some structure.

From an outsider perspective, it can sound boring, but it works. It feels right.

3.

Navigating Non-monogamy

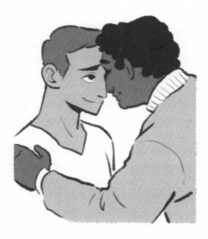

....

I've always been one of those girls who likes to date. There are a lot of words for women like me—ladies who fall in love easily, enjoy sex, and aren't set on finding "the one"—and none of them are nice.

I was raised to be confident, to make my own way in the world and live my dreams and proudly ride the reading rainbow, etcetera, etcetera. But whenever I find myself pursuing multiple people, there's this tinny voice in my brain that says one word: slut, slut, slut.

Every serious relationship I've ever been in has involved freak-outs over monogamy issues. A few weeks, months, or years in, a drumbeat starts in me. Am I really going to sleep with just this guy for the rest of my life? I think about all of the great people in the world. I dwell on the things that are missing from our relationship. I contemplate all the intense, unique connections that could be possible in my life. I fixate on how my boyfriend is completely annoying sometimes and no one is "made for each other." I feel trapped, like my life path is shrinking down to one small door. The tension rises in me. This, in the past, has led to me cheating. Or becoming so obsessed with the idea of being with someone else that I abandon my relationship and we break up.

Onward and upward. Around and around.

My parents' generation did a solid job of opening up opportunities for women. But reforms in the home and workplace haven't breached the central idea that women should seek monogamy. The idea of relationships as a white knight saving a damsel has been disbanded, but there have been few positive models to replace that fairy tale narrative.

There's still this core belief in our society that while people will date around while they're young, a liberated gal like me will eventually find a husband and settle down. And if that doesn't work—if one of us succumbs to our internal drumbeat and has sex with someone else—the proper thing to do is to get divorced and go in search of new soul mates.

This brought me to the big questions that kept me up at night as I turned 25 and hit the two-year mark in my relationship with Carl. He's smart. He's funny. He's curious about the world. And he loved me. But there was this cloud of anxiety, this nagging idea: Is monogamy necessary? Is it for me? And how the hell do people have sex with one person for 50 years and still be happy?

While I've felt inclined toward non-monogamy, I didn't want to smash my relationship to bits figuring out the logistics. Despite reading a couple books on the topic, the stakes of jumping in to non-monogamy felt impossibly high. What if I honestly and intentionally slept with someone else and it ruined my relationship with my boyfriend forever?

I desperately wanted straight-up advice on the pitfalls and long-term viability of open relationships from people who have already drawn out the learning curve of ethical non-monogamous relationships. Talking to several dozen people in various types of open relationships, I learned a lot. Mostly, I learned that open relationships aren't an unachievable fantasy. Thousands of Americans have successful short-term and long-term open relationships; most of them just don't talk about their private lives very publicly. Open relationships aren't easy and they're not for everybody. If Carl and I wanted to be non-monogamous, we would have to be game for doing the hard work of being more honest and less jealous than comes naturally, for deeply analyzing our intentions, and for being outspoken about what we want sexually.

Carl and I decided we were up for that complicated work, at least for a while to see how it worked for us. It involved lots of emotional work and lots of conversation—not just between Carl and me, but between us and anyone else we slept with. Luckily, as much as we were making up what our relationship looked like as we went along, many people have experience with open relationships and shared their logistical wisdom.

Open relationships involve a lot of letting go. But, overall, I think non-monogamy can be a fun, positive part of my relationship with my boyfriend—a force that makes our relationship better, not a threat that destroys it.

The Details

First off, it turns out there are a bunch of different ways to have an open relationship. Here is a short list of some I have encountered:

• A guy who has no single, steady girlfriend, but has emotional and sexual relationships with multiple people— some of whom are good friends who stick around his life for a long time, some are relative strangers who he sees rarely or only once.

• A woman who has a "primary" girlfriend she has dated for years and lives with during the week and a boyfriend she sleeps with on weekends.

• A genderqueer couple that is almost entirely monogamous, except they sometimes have sex with other people if one of them is out of town.

• A man who is monogamous with his girlfriend, but she's not into kinky sex, so he occasionally sees another woman with whom he has a dominant/submissive relationship.

• A male-female couple that every once in a while invites another woman over for sex.

• A married gay couple who share the same third partner as a joint boyfriend.

• A male-female couple who are committed to each other long-term but go on dates with other people—sometimes alone, sometimes as a double date—and often have sex with those other partners either alone or together.

• A married male-female couple who each have a separate girlfriend and boyfriend, respectively, that they are emotionally and sexually involved with long-term.

Within all these relationships, many couples switch occasionally between being monogamous or non-monogamous, depending on how they're feeling and what's going on with the relationship. When they need to focus on their primary relationship, some people end their other relationships—sometimes for good, sometimes just temporarily. Other people stick consistently with the same non-monogamous arrangements for years and years.

People hear "open relationship" and they often think: "Having sex with lots of people all the time! Orgies, woohoo!" But in reality, sex is just one part of a giant change in the way you approach dating.

The foundation of open relationships is a simple idea: One person can't be a 100 percent perfect partner for any other person. Nor should we expect them to be. Hoping your boyfriend or girlfriend will fit unrealistic expectations of perfection is only going to lead to frustration, disappointment, and resentment. Under this idea, attraction to multiple people is a positive, honest, wholesome part of someone's life, rather than an inherently nasty, negative urge to "cheat."

One Portlander named Mary who has been in an open relationship for fifteen years summed up her core philosophy beautifully:

> "Being in love is not enough. There's this cultural idea that being in love can overcome all obstacles— that's just not true. Love is valuable and worth fighting for, but not worth being miserable for years. If you're not happy in your relationship, something needs to change."

A lot of people seek open relationships after seeing adherence to monogamy wreck havoc on friends or family. Allena, a sex activist in Seattle, told me the story of her grandma, who'd been married to her grandpa for 70 years when he died at age 100. "She said he was a 'good provider,' but a terrible husband," says Allena. "I knew what that meant. We were raised to be looking for 'the one.' This makes me gag. If you're not looking around for the one, you don't have to waste your life."

It's hard to see how much our lives are built around the presumption of "the one" love until you start to consider the logistics of being ethically non-monogamous (plenty of people—ahem, Rush Limbaugh—are *unethically* non-monogamous). Creating a life that includes multiple partners means rethinking our entire approach to love, sex, and relationships. It means doing scary things like recognizing where our partners fall short for us and defining for ourselves what loyalty and betrayal mean. It means talking often about who you're attracted to and what makes you insecure. It means drawing up your own map for what makes your relationships special.

People always wonder about "the rules" for open relationships, but people I interviewed universally said they don't micromanage their relationships with a long list of rules. Instead, their relationships are built around basic principles and general ideas.

Allena, for example, has one rule: "No surprises."

Lucy, a twentysomething born and raised in Brooklyn, had only one rule with her long-term non-monogamous boyfriend: "Be Classy." That covers everything from no-texting-one-person-while-you're-with-another to "yes, of course wash the sheets between partners."

There's a lot of debate over whether people are born monogamous or whether our biology is geared toward having relationships with multiple people. The current thinking is that there's a lot in history to suggest that humans are naturally inclined toward non-monogamy and it's our cultural institutions—like churches and U.S. tax law—that contain those impulses by stressing monogamy. Even if we're not built for monogamy, many people decide it's a better personal choice for them. Of course, the problem is that many people don't realize there is a choice at all.

20 Lessons From People in Open Relationships
1. **It's high time to invent a word other than "boyfriend."**

    Everyone knows what "boyfriend" means and what "wife" means. But how do you tell your friends about your wife's boyfriend?

    One problem with non-monogamy is there's no good vocabulary to describe it. There's a world of relationships between "boyfriend" (which implies monogamy) and "friend" (which implies you two aren't getting it on). Wrapped up in this lack of lexicon is a deeply engrained societal belief that one-man-one-woman is the *only* way for a relationship to work and that all relationships should have the end goal of long-term monogamy.

There are all sorts of terms people use for their not-monogamous partners, but some are awkward and you should use what feels best to you. Among these words is "polyamorous"—someone who naturally wants multiple loving partnerships and sexual relationships. There's also "solo-poly"—someone who likes to have steady partnerships, but goes it alone with multiple relationships. Many people who have a steady, long-term partner describe that main relationship as their "primary" partner and as other relationships as "secondary" partnerships.

But people tend to make up whatever title they think works for their not-boyfriend, not-husband partners. Some titles people use in real life include: partner, lover, boo, date, person I'm dating, secondary partner, boyfriend or girlfriend, friend, friend with benefits, sweetie, ladyfriend, guy on the side. None are perfect, so use whatever feels right.

2. **Monogamy isn't for everybody.**
   It can take a while to wrap your brain around the idea that there's really nothing "wrong" or amoral about non-monogamy. Getting over the shame we have around "sluts" and "cheaters" is a big job. So work on that.

   Meanwhile, try to figure out whether you actually want to be in an open relationship. Many people sort through this by writing, talking, and using their imaginations.

   Write out a list of what you absolutely need in a long-term partner and, if you have a current partner, how they meet those needs (or don't). Do you want a partner who's an adventure companion? Someone who cares about your work? Someone to raise kids with? Someone for kinky sex? What needs must be filled by your partner and which could someone else conceivable fill?

   Talk about open relationships and pick out what you think are good ideas. Susan, who grew up fundamentalist Christian and married her husband when they were just shy of twenty, started listening to sex advice columnist Dan Savage's *Savage Love* podcast and found she related to some of the people who called in with questions about polyamory. She and her husband talked about those examples and realized they could imagine their own life being like that. Another married couple in Boston wasn't sure about opening up, so they attended a potluck hosted by a polyamory group and talked with people about their relationships—they took on some ideas as models and nixed others they didn't like (in their case: no group sex, but frequent individual dates).

You need to sort out how you feel about having multiple sexual relationships. Sit and imagine what your life would be like if you had sex with more than one person in a year. Does that sound like something you want to do, or not? What would your reaction be if your boyfriend told you he kissed someone, had a crush on someone, or fucked someone? If your gut says one of these situations makes you queasy, that might be a boundary for you. It might wind up that your boundaries exclude everything except sex with one person for the rest of your life—but they might not.

3. **Be more honest.**
Your relationships can look however you want them to look. But you have to honest about what you want. Instead of dismissing ideas that make you nervous, try to pinpoint exactly what makes you nervous—are you insecure that your partner would find someone more attractive than you? Are you worried that having sex with multiple people would decrease your intimacy with one-on-one relationships? These kinds of fears are totally valid, but you've got to articulate them to yourself before you and your partners can actually deal with them.

When people in open relationships talked to me about what works, two big words keep coming up: Honesty and intention. Non-monogamy requires making intentional relationships, not slipping into relationships by default or without thinking through the consequences. And they require being honest with everyone involved—starting with yourself—to an extent that most people find difficult at first.

4. **Tell your partner that you want an open relationship.**

This seems obvious, but a lot of people never take the scary plunge of telling their partners that they want to be non-monogamous.

Elaine, a 46 year-old-mother living in Berkeley, went through two marriages before she finally spit out the words. The third time around, she decided to be extremely honest.

"I finally laid my cards on the table: 'I need to be in relationships with many people, not just one,'" says Elaine. "I expected him to run screaming, but he said, 'No, that's great.'"

Honesty is a constant process. It's the kind of work that never stops. It entails talking, talking, and more talking.

If you've already got a long-term partner and you've come to the conclusion that you want to be non-monogamous, that's totally a possibility. Not every couple lands on common ground together, but some do. Getting on the same page together requires a lot of conversation. Take heart in knowing that thousands of people have done this before—they just usually keep it quiet when it works well.

You can ease into the conversation by testing the waters of their reaction to non-monogamy issues in general. Several people I met with, started this conversation by mentioning that they saw a TV show about polyamory or talked with a friend about open relationships.

After talking about issues hypothetically, many couples talk about their own thoughts on monogamy. Talk about what you would want and desire from other people and define your boundaries. Finally—often weeks or months later—act on the theories by flirting with others or asking them out.

5. **Don't cheat—talk.**

Talking over non-monogamy is exponentially more difficult for partners that don't trust each other. Waiting until someone cheats and then trying to open up the relationship is difficult, say people who've walked through that fire. It's not impossible, but couples that come to a decision to start an open relationship together are building trust together, rather than wading through betrayal retroactively.

Darren, a programmer in the Bay Area, had been married for a few years before his wife confessed to cheating and said she wanted an open relationship. He was devastated, but decided that the most important thing in his life was staying in his marriage and raising his daughter with his wife, so he's been willing to work through the difficult opening-up process.

"I knew, obviously, our marriage was going to change, but was it going to change beyond recognition? Will we still be intimate? Will we still have sex regularly?" fretted Darren. A year into the open relationship, it was still hard. Darren still felt angry at his wife and has trouble trusting her. But all the conversations have made their relationship more transparent—they still have problems, but at least they know what the problems are and they're out in the open.

6. **Be frank about what your relationship looks like.**
So is this a long-term relationship? A once-a-month sleepover? A date-whenever-my-boyfriend-is-busy arrangement? People need to be on the same page about what a relationship is going to look like, otherwise disappointment and disagreement is inevitable.

Conflicts arrive in open relationships when people feel like a new idea is sprung on them at the last minute, or undertaken without talking about it together first. If you're going on a date with someone and think you'll have sex, don't tell you're partner you're expecting just to hold hands.

If you're not in a long-term relationship already or are dating multiple people casually, decide how to bring up what you want and need and how intimate to get with partners conversationally. You don't have to soul search with a one-night stand, but if you're dating someone new, you've got to actually say out loud what you want and expect, not hope they'll infer your intentions by the way you kiss them. It also means clueing them into other relationships you have going on.

A friend of mine told me that a woman he went on dates with occasionally said to him, "Think of me as your back-pocket girl."

"I have no idea what that means," he replied. "I need a number."

"Twice a month?" she offered. Deal.

Lots of non-monogamous people use dating websites because it's handy to spell out specifically what their personal situations are before they sit down for a drink with someone new. In 2012, many folks recommended the website OkCupid.com, which has a lot of people in open relationships as users and lets people spell out exactly what kind of set-up they're hoping for on new dates.

7. Say yes only when you mean yes.

For better or worse, we're a species that's easily talked into things. If someone feels manipulated into a relationship situation they're not okay with or not given a safe, honest chance to say "no" to, things are going to get explosive at some point (or, perhaps worse, things will get sulky and sullen for a long time).

A lot of people say it's hard to figure out how to say yes and how to say no to partners' ideas. You want to be open-minded and up for adventures, but you also don't want to wind up getting your heart torn apart by signing off on something you're actually not okay with.

So take it slow. People have a tendency to jump the gun on sex. The key finding from long-term non-monogamous folks is that conversation prevents meltdown. You have to build trust and solid communication with every new partner, plus keep your old partners in the loop on your actions and feelings.

Lots of couples deal with "saying yes" by giving each other "veto power" on whether or not it's okay to date a specific person.

Another good idea: Waiting 24 hours before making decisions on any new idea your partner brings up. Think it over and you'll likely know more solidly how you feel. In the same vein, one couple established a "G-chat moratorium" after conversations over Google's instant message platform led to stilted yes's and petulant no's—now they talk about all relationship ideas face-to-face.

Worst-case scenario is you jump into bed with someone and the experience brings up issues that should have been discussed *before* all the clothes came off.

Evan, a dancing instructor, related the story of dating woman who suggested having a threesome with her husband. The husband seemed to be okay with it, but the three didn't sit down and talk about the idea together. In the midst of the threesome, the husband had an emotional breakdown.

"I ended up being a naked marriage counselor," laments Evan.

8. Brace yourself for getting turned down.

It's rare to find two people who want the same kind of arrangement. Plus, needs change over time. Someone who wants an occasional-lover in October may realize they want a long-term boyfriend by November.

It seems that straight men with girlfriends have an especially hard time finding women who are on-board for being the secondary partner or side-girl. That's unfortunate, though not surprising, given societal norms paint men as likely to cheat and lie. But regardless of gender and orientation, people have trouble finding partners who are of like mind about monogamy. Many times, people who think they'd be down for open relationships find they're surprisingly possessive, jealous, or a fan of simplicity.

9. Note that there are only 24 hours in each day.

The sad fact is that non-monogamy means dividing that time between more people.

A lot of people balance schedules by agreeing to a rough amount of time they'll spend with each partner. Whether it's one sleepover night a week, "only when I'm out of town," or weekends with one person and weekdays with another, people work out all sorts of approximately set time schedules.

It's good to let partners know as far in advance as possible when you'll be able to see them and when you have other dates scheduled. Just a day or two will do for many people, but the trick is to tell partners your plans as soon as *you* know, otherwise it can seem like you're being deceitful. Planning ahead shows a respect for partners' time, plus it gives them a chance to line up other activities.

A lot of people find it's smart to keep busy while their partners are on dates, otherwise they can get lonely and start to dwell on how much fun the other person must be having. Call up friends, call up a crush, schedule a work-party; use the time without an available partner to live your own life.

As of 2012, a lot of people used Google calendars to maneuver around multiple lovers' schedules. Google's shared-calendars system allows users to invite multiple people to view whatever dates they enter. Plus, you can color code. Excellent.

10. **Consider kissing and telling.**

The gory details: Some people love 'em, some people hate 'em.

It's important to figure out how much you want to know about what your partner is up to. A handful of people really don't want to know what their partners are doing with other people—a "don't ask, don't tell" policy. But most people in open relationships want to know at least some info about their partners' other sex lives. Some people want to know all the graphic sexual details, some people just want to know the names of other people their partners are sleeping with. Open relationships seem to be more stable when everyone involved long-term knows each other at least a little.

Part of what's good about kissing-and-telling is that jealousy can be born from feeling left out of the excitement of other relationships. Humans are story-making machines and pretty much everybody finds themselves imagining what their partners are up to in bed with other people. That drives some people crazy. Sharing details about what sex and dates are like with other people can cut down on our brain's terrible imaginary stories.

Bay Area husband and wife Josh and Michelle describe themselves as not-jealous people, but they still tell each other pretty much all of the graphic details from their dates. Otherwise, says Michelle, "You can come to very drastic conclusions. I like getting to know how much fun he had, rather than sitting at home *wondering* how much fun he had."

11. **Meet your partner's other partners.**

Meet your partner's other partners in person, on your own, without your partner around as intermediary. Get a sandwich. Get a drink. Keep it low-key, low-pressure, and friendly. Getting to know them as a person can help dissolve feelings of jealousy and intimidation.

Taking it up a major notch, some people recommend, at some point, having sex with a third person together— it can help cut down on your imagination running wild to actually see your partner with another person. That's definitely not for everyone, but some people say it has helped them deal with jealousy a lot.

Some people develop good relationships with their partner's other people.

"My boyfriend bakes my husband cakes," says Susan, the Seattle former-fundamentalist. That's clearly an absurdly best-case scenario. Sometimes it doesn't work out so well.

Tyler is a life-long non-monogamist and has a rule that her partner can't date any of their mutual friends, preferring to keep sexual relationships and trusted friendships separate. One time she bent the "no friends" rule, okaying her partner's desire to hook up regularly with one of their close friends. That situation ended bitterly, when Tyler felt like the friend was getting too romantic and driving a wedge between the couple.

12. **Only have safe sex.**

Condoms are annoying, birth control is a hassle, STD tests are expensive. But you know what's worse than all three combined? Giving an STD to someone you love.

Relentlessly practicing safer sex is a must for open relationships because having sex with numerous people puts you at higher risk for getting an STD. In addition to always using condoms and birth control if you're fooling around with multiple people, it's smart to get an STD test every six months or anytime you're about to start having sex with a new person. As a decent human being, you're contractually obligated to talk about STDs and pregnancy before you have sex with someone. Before there's any genital-to-genital action, offer up your own status, talk about what method of birth control you guys are using, and ask if they have any diseases you should know about. It can suck being the person who brings up these issues, especially if you have an STD and know that discussing it could stop your romance in its tracks. But don't you dare skip that conversation and burn yourself with a lifetime of guilt (or a lifetime of herpes).

13. **Come out to important people.**

Myself and others have found that the hard truth of the matter is that no matter how much some people love you, they will react negatively to your open relationship. A lot of peoples' only experience with open relationships is as a last-ditch effort of couples easing into break-up, or as a manipulative justification to cheat.

There are a lot of negative narratives built around people who have multiple romantic relationships: You're a slut, you're using people for sex, you're a heartbreaker, you're anti-romantic. For these reasons, most people in non-monogamous relationships are careful about whom they tell the details of their relationships. A lot of people compare the process of telling their family and close friends about their non-monogamy as similar to "coming out" as queer.

Some heart-on-their-sleeves people who live in more tolerant places see non-monogamy as no big deal and talk about it with strangers and coworkers. But most people in long-term open relationships tell only close friends or are only "out" in specific circles. If people don't know you're in an open relationship, they'll assume you're monogamous and off-limits. A lot of people can describe awkward moments where friends or acquaintances saw them on a date and thought they were cheating. Having your relationship situation known deters these negative assumptions and also lets people know you're potentially looking for new partners.

If you're coming out to family and friends, be straightforward about your relationship, but hold off on sharing all the juicy details—it can come off as bragging, and a lot of people don't really want to know your exploits.

Brandon, a Seattleite who's married and shares a long-term boyfriend with his husband, had some trouble when he told his mom he wanted to bring both guys home for Thanksgiving.

"My poor mother, I've had to come out to her three times: First as an atheist, then as gay man, then as open," says Brandon. His mother was worried about him being promiscuous and at risk for HIV, but over time she's become more okay with her son's relationships, says Brandon.

When kids are older, parents in open relationships usually clue them into their multiple relationships depending on how they talk with the kids about other touchy topics around sex and dating.

Elaine, the thrice-married mom in Berkeley, goes on regular dates and occasional trips with another guy. After a year maintaining both her marriage and the side-relationship, she felt confident and comfortable enough with it to be honest about the situation with her teenage kids. But they don't want to hear about it.

"I sat the kids down and explained to them that [my husband and I] believe this is okay, that our boyfriend is part of our life. I said, 'This might be uncomfortable for you,' but I wanted to have them talk back to us about it. My son said basically, 'That's okay, but I don't want it in my face.' My fifteen-year-old daughter was like, 'Okay, that's interesting.'"

Some parents tell their kids the essentials and keep their dating life outside of the house and relatively out of sight; other parents introduce their kids to their other partners. What works well seems to depend on how healthy and stable the relationships themselves are and how the parents relate to their kids to begin with.

14. Know your problems.

I tend to be a liar by omission. I don't go wandering around telling my boyfriend bold untruths, but I bite my tongue when I'm feeling something I know they wouldn't like. With long-term partners, those quiet complaints build into a volcano of resentment that eventually erupts. And that gets messy.

That's why honesty is a process, a practice. I've started actively working to tell my partners things that I can feel myself shoveling into that resentment volcano.

Everyone has disagreements and complicated feelings, but open relationships raise the stakes on a lot of issues, accelerating those potential eruptions. For non-monogamous relationships to work without anyone getting burned, the partners have to be more honest and work harder to recognize and address problems than in monogamous relationships. So long-term non-monogamous people have developed strategies to articulate inevitable relationship problems.

People in successful open relationships make voicing problems an integral part of their relationship, rather than something that only happens after someone feels irreparably hurt or stomped on. If no one is voicing complaints, that means someone—maybe you—is doing what I do and stockpiling an explosive reserve of resentment. The strength of the partnership is how they deal with this tough stuff.

This sounds hokey, but one way a lot of partners work on knowing their problems is to have a designated time when someone can easily raise a complaint. Some people make sure to check-in and debrief after every date with a new person. One Boston couple—whose approach to complaints is complicated by them also being in a dominant-submissive relationship—has a strategy where either person can declare "free speech time" and bring up concerns that the other person has to actively try not to judge or dismiss.

Some of the best honesty strategies come from people who have been through hell. Darren, the Bay Area programmer whose marriage opened up after his wife cheated on him, has to deal with a lot of issues of anger and betrayal. When arguments get heated and personal, he or his wife calls a time out—they drop the argument and resume it after a day, when they've had time to think about it. They've also actively worked on verbalizing exactly what they're feeling, rather than relying on body language. If things are too difficult to say to each other aloud, they say them first to friends or write it out in an email.

"I've got a big inbox of drafts," jokes Darren. Surprisingly, even after going through the hell of dealing with the wife's affair, Darren says that if he were to choose, he wouldn't go back to monogamy. The high stakes of polyamory have helped his wife and him talk about their problems, rather than brushing them under the rug.

"We now have very defined, solvable problems," he says. "They're quite big, but they're clearly defined."

15. Don't be a jerk when you fall crazy in love.

There's this chemical thing that happens to your brain when you're excited about someone new. What we call "having a crush" could more accurately be called "going crazy on drugs."

In the first little while—days, weeks, months—that you're attracted to someone new, your brain floods with dopamine and serotonin. That contributes to a phenomena that people in open relationships often call "new relationship energy"—the love-drunk feeling of delight when you're with someone new. The world can disappear. And while that's awesome, it can be trouble if you're supposed to be a responsible and attentive lover to someone else, too.

Falling crazy in love can make you kind of a jerk to your current partners. That doesn't mean you shouldn't revel in the feeling, but you should be aware that you might be acting like an idiot.

People in successful open relationships try to appreciate new relationship energy for what it's worth: It can make you super horny, really happy, and less stressed. But you also have to recognize that your brain is not functioning rationally and not to make any drastic life choices (like, say, breaking up or moving across the country) under these dopamine-flooded conditions.

16. Investigate your jealousy.

I thought jealousy would be the big problem for open relationships. Two people sleeping with the same person is the point of conflict for roughly every piece of literature in the canon.

But people in open relationships say "jealousy" is too vague of a term—what I think of as jealous is really a symptom that arises from a bunch of different problems. To figure out why you're feeling jealous, you have to dissect exactly what fears and behaviors are at its root.

One issue that's often at the root of jealousy is lack of trust. People get jealous when they feel like their partners are lying to them or withholding their true feelings. Someone can lie about flirting with a friend at a party and it can provoke the same intensity of jealousy as actually having sex with that friend, because if the action is covert, both are a violation of trust. On the flip side, people say they're surprised at how calm they are about big scary actions when there's a solid foundation of trust.

"At the beginning, the thought of my wife with another man made me want to go incredible Hulk on them," said one married Californian. "Now, I know I'll see her when she gets back."

17. Romance can hurt.

Another problem that leads to jealousy is when people want more from a relationship than someone can give. Open relationships can be a delicate balance between the time, lust, and needs of all the people involved. Usually, it's a "secondary" partner who winds up feeling hurt or resentful because they're never going to be their partner's number-one-lover. Discussing those expectations and making each relationship valuable in its own way is essential.

On the flip side, plenty of "primary" partners get nervous when they feel like their partner is creating a serious relationship on the side. A lot of people say they actually get more jealous about their partner's romantic, emotional connections with other people than them having sex. Hooking up with someone during a lunch break can seem like a smaller deal than receiving a heartfelt letter and flowers, because the latter could feel like an infringement on what's "special" about that primary relationship.

Romance can threaten the intimacy of a primary relationship, so keep a weather eye focused on your own actions and intentions as well as your partners'.

18. **Keep your relationships special.**

So how is your husband different than your boyfriend if you are in love with both of them and have sex with both of them? Ah. That's the somewhat unquantifiable part of open relationships and it gets back to the "specialness" that's a big part of jealousy.

For monogamous relationships, the clear demarcation between what type of relationship you have with someone is whether or not you're having sex. But non-monogamous people have to define for themselves what the difference is between their various relationships. Some of those definable lines are obvious behaviors, and some of them are completely inexplicable feelings that one relationship is more intimate and central to your life than another.

One thing is for sure: creating mutual expectations around time, emotional and sexual intimacy, and decision-making is tough.

Some people do that by saying they only "love" their primary partners. But love is a vague term that can mean different things to different people.

More often, people in open relationships express the difference between relationships via specific behaviors. For example, some people define their relationships by spending significantly more time with one partner than another. Some people have certain sex acts that they reserve for one partner. Some people decide to include secondary partners in on big life-plan "family issues" like career changes, where to live, whether to get married, or whether to have kids, while a lot of people see those things as the sort of conversations they have just with one partner.

19. **Kids are a time-suck.**

There's a joke about open relationships: "They work, until you have kids."

Having children adds a new layer to time-management in open relationships. But some people manage to have kids and be non-monogamous.

Definitely a lot of people I talked to backed off from their non-primary relationships when they had young children. Babies gobble up free time like date-killing black holes; running out for a date doesn't seem so appealing when you were up all night with a crying baby. Having a child also adds a level of negotiation to dating multiple people, since someone has to stay home with the kid (or pay for the babysitter). Rather than having couples be able to head their separate ways on different dates, people with kids often either have to trade off nights, or do more dates together, like, for example, starting out the night with a group playing boardgames until one parent peels off with a date while the other keeps track of their kid.

A lot of people wind up having more at-home dates. One non-monogamous woman in Portland said her relationship with her boyfriend involved less sex after she had a child, but the pair still hung out regularly.

"We used to have sex a lot, but we haven't been very often since I've had a baby. It's been a lot more difficult to get time alone," she says. "Now we have 'old married lesbian dates'—getting take out and watching *MASH*."

20. Be confident that you are awesome.

Carrying on multiple relationships can easily lead to feeling competitive. Many people find this innate urge to ask, "Who's do you like fucking better? Who's prettier? Who's smarter?" Nipping that in the bud is a Sisyphean task, but it helps to recognize that each person in the relationship has wonderful and valuable traits. Appreciating the differences between partners helps people recognize what's unique and good about each.

Last Thoughts

I expected that open relationships would be much more complicated and messy than monogamous relationships. But in talking to people and in my own relationship, I found that non-monogamy can create a good kind of complication. Keeping multiple people on the same page expectation-wise means having to engage in lots of conversation together about the tough, awkward stuff we usually prefer to clam up about.

Carl and I were in an open relationship for about a year-and-a-half. At first we were terrified and excited. It felt like the whole paradigm of our relationship had changed. Suddenly, I could flirt with people and not feel bad about it. I could tell him when I had a crush on someone and we'd laugh about it together. I could breathe much more easily than I ever had before. When we started going on dates with other people, I felt like we were embarking on that scene at the end of *Indiana Jones and the Last Crusade*, where he steps out over a vast crevasse and miraculously finds a bridge. Every small step forward felt like a leap of faith. When our steps kept falling on solid ground after a thrilling adventure like sleeping over at other peoples' houses, I was overjoyed. Our open relationship made me feel extremely lucky and loved.

I was surprised to find that people felt stable in a diverse variety of relationship types. It seems like every person I meet in an open relationship had a different set-up—there's no magic number of partners or rules about number of dates per week that are clearly the best. Instead, people feel great or terrible in myriad arrangements. Open relationships that work well for all involved universally hinge on how the people involved deal with large, deep issues of honesty, intention, and trust. It comes back to practicing those good habits, where the better road is often the one that's harder in the short term.

I feel like non-monogamy is a good and necessary part of my life for as far out to the horizon as I can see. But non-monogamy is a fluid, changing thing. So far, the ideal set-up for me is having a stable, wonderful boyfriend with whom I build a life, and also occasionally having fun with a lover-on-the-side, too. Maybe in the future I'll want to date another couple with a boyfriend, or join a polyamorous board-game sex-party group, or—gasp—feel like being sexual with only one person for years and years. We'll see. I feel good about having options.

I started talking to people in open relationships feeling like a broken freak for being attracted to different people all the time and feeling driven to cheat on partners. Meeting dozens of people who face attraction and see it as a positive thing, not something to fear, was rather mind-blowing. It has taken me some serious time to come around to the idea that feeling attracted to lots of people in my life can be a good thing, not something that's going to doom all my relationships to fail. Additionally, whether we choose non-monogamy or not, the skills it develops for honesty and communication strengthen all relationships and can reveal weaker areas that need work much faster than monogamous relationships.

The core philosophy behind open relationships is that sex and love between numerous people creates positive interactions—the dark, negative side of sex is where people feel unloved and unattractive. Sex shouldn't be a competitive sport, but a beneficial arrangement where everyone involved feels sexier, more fulfilled, and more excited about their lives.

Tristan Taormino

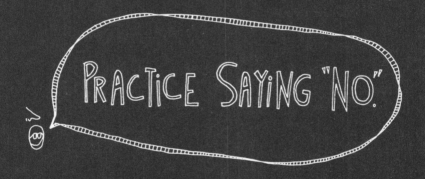

Practice Saying "No."

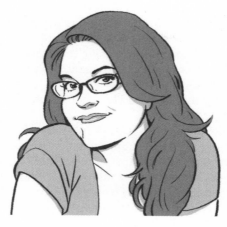

Tristan Taormino is well-known for her work as a feminist pornographer and prolific sex writer, but I first found out about her when I got an angry phone call from a student at Oregon State University. I was a reporter for a Portland alt-weekly and the call was from a sex-positive student group who had invited Taormino to give a talk on "Claiming Your Sexual Power." A week before the event, school administrators balked on paying the speaking fee of a "self-described pornographer" and cancelled the event, leading to uproar. I interviewed Tristan about the debacle and, in contrast to the university administrators, found her very worth listening to.

Tristan is straightforward about sex in a refreshing way. She built a career out of offering practical, unabashed advice about the kinds of bedroom acts that most people would rarely whisper to their friends about. She promotes making feminist porn as a way to change the media landscape around sex and relationships. While most Americans watch porn, it's not a form of media we critique and discuss as openly as, say, network television. But the images and relationships we see in porn undoubtedly shape our ideas of our bodies and our sexualities. Tristan walks the talk on the idea that if we're serious about being sex positive and body positive, we should work to create equitable and honest sexual relationships both on and off-screen.

A year later, her writing became personally important to me. When I started thinking that my boyfriend and I should be in an open relationship. I read her great book on logistics and thinking behind non-monogamy, Opening Up. It's one of the few books about relationships that has made me feel understood rather than crazy. I talked with Taormino one afternoon in a Portland hotel lobby after I attended her sold-out workshop on open relationships.

No, There's No Script For Relationships

My first serious girlfriend was in college; she was older than me. When she graduated, she moved to LA. We had a discussion that now we were going to be long distance and only see each other every couple months, shouldn't we have an open relationship?

In theory that seemed like a good idea at the time. In practice, it was a disaster.

I wasn't opposed to it. It didn't strike fear in me the moment she brought it up. I'm a practical person. I was like, "Listen, we're going to be apart and we're in our twenties, it doesn't seem like we should wait forever for each other." I had already experienced my own awakening in terms of my queer identity, so I was used to thinking outside of the box in that way.

It made sense: If all of these things are possible in sex, then all of these things must be possible in relationships, too. We don't have to stick to a script, there's no better way or more normal way to do this. There are options.

But we didn't negotiate well. For that school year, we were in an open relationship and we both saw other people. I had flings with people. She had a relationship with someone who was still in the picture when I came to see her the next summer. And then we were in this position like: What do we do now? Things disintegrated from there, though she did stop seeing the woman temporarily, it just didn't work.

I have to cut myself some slack; I was twenty. I couldn't figure out until my late twenties what I wanted and what I needed. What were my deal breakers and what was available for compromise?

I did the best that I could, but it wasn't very good.

Last night, this couple came up to me after the workshop. They waited until the end, which usually means they have something to ask me that they don't want anyone to overhear. They're married, they seemed to be in their twenties, and he said he's come to this place where he thinks he's polyamorous. And she's monogamous, so she was like, "I don't think this is my ideal relationship." And I thought, what is that?

"The ideal relationship." It's so abstract. No one has an ideal relationship with anyone, but we still hang on to this idea that there is such a thing. Let's reframe it. Could he be an ideal partner for you? Is he meeting your needs? Are you meeting his? Rather than, does this look like you thought your marriage would look when you were twelve?

Casual Sex Shouldn't Be Casual

People talk about casual sex as sex without love or emotional attachment. Those words don't mean a whole lot. "Casual" implies a lack of intention and consciousness. Like: I'm wearing sweat pants, I'm having sex with you.

You could have the most deep emotional connection with someone that you just met and you could know and fuck someone for years and never have that intense of a connection as you had with this other person. The ways that we measure intimacy or connection are individual for people.

There's not even a good phrase for having sex when you don't want to pursue commitment or a relationship with a capital R. Monogamy has a pretty strong grip on our world. It's so ingrained in how we think about relationships that much of it goes unexamined.

Even I Can Be Monogamous Sometimes

Most of my relationships have not been monogamous in some form or another, but I can think of one or two that have been monogamous. Right now, my Colten and I are mono-non-mono. I'm monogamous and Colten is not monogamous.

For me, figuring out whether to be monogamous is a conscious discussion of, "Where am I at in my life right now? What do I need? What do I want? What does the other person need, what do they want, what feels right for this interaction?"

In one of my monogamous relationships, I was going through a lot of shit in my life. My father had just died. I needed a sense of stability and security and in my 24-year-old brain, I'm thinking monogamy is stable and secure—which now I would argue that it's not.

Colten and I are gay married and we've been non-monogamous since the beginning. We've had, wow, a lot of different styles. First off, we were polyamorous and we were not each other's primary partners—we each had other primary partners. Then we became primary partners and still had other partners. Then we had a period where we did partnered non-monogamy, where we were the primary couple and we had sex play on the side, but we did it all together, so we were like a package deal and always had a third or a fourth person. That lasted many years. For me, I'm in a place right now where I want this one person and I don't have time or energy for anything else. My work is important to me, so that comes first. I have intense friendships—that are not romantic or sexual—with people that I spend a lot of time on, so I don't feel like there's room for other people, and there's not a desire driving it.

Getting involved with other people takes time, energy, and work and I'm just not up for it right now.

Practice Saying "No."
I have been someone in the past who, when my partner asks if they can do something, my automatic kneejerk reaction is yes. I say it quickly and I don't really evaluate the situation.

I have to consciously tell myself: Even if this feels 100 percent good, let me think about it overnight, or give me a day to think about it. That way I can check in with myself and think, "Okay, do I have any feelings about this at all?"

My tendency is to jump to yes and then later go, wait a second, I should have thought through this, I should have set a couple more boundaries or made something more clear, but instead I'm so gung ho to get to yes that I don't take into account my own feelings.

Part of leaning how to be non-monogamous is trial and error and part of it is listening to my own instincts. When I think about my partner fucking one of my friends, my body just tells me that's not cool. I feel tense in my stomach, like anxiety. Whereas if I think of my partner fucking someone he met at the class last night, my instincts don't tell me that's a bad idea. There's no red flag for me.

So much of this is listening to your inner voice; listening to what your instincts tell you. If your instincts tell you this is going to be trouble, it is.

ERiKA MOEN

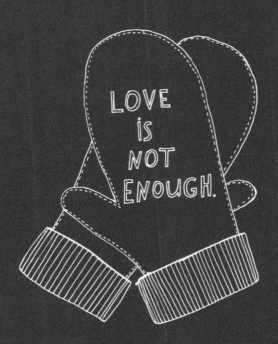

LOVE
iS
NOT
ENOUGH.

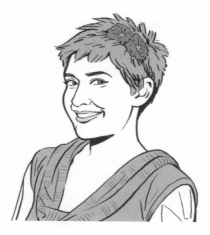

Erika Moen has a hilarious job: The 30-year-old cartoonist spends most of her days drawing a comics series about the ins-and-outs of sex toys. Her work, including a long-running autobiographical comic called DAR, paints a portrait of a life full of creative friends and great sex. But for a feminist, queer, sex-positive cartoonist, Moen is surprisingly conservative in her relationships. When we met for burritos in the basement of her Portland studio, Moen gushed about being madly in love with her husband, Matt, with whom she was in a long-distance, monogamous relationship for over three years. Recently, they have dabbled in non-monogamy, but after five years of marriage, still feel like they're in "storybook love."

Love Is Not Enough

I didn't really date in high school. I felt like a late bloomer. I knew other girls knew how to masturbate and have orgasms and I couldn't figure that shit out at all. I didn't have real romantic relationships; I had compulsive crushes on guys. I would choose them and fixate on them and desperately want to be loved back. It wasn't really fun.

But simultaneous to this, I had my best friend, a lady. We had a close, intimate, somewhat physical relationship with each other. And we'd sleep together at each other's houses a lot. There was sexual energy and sexual experimentation, but it didn't occur to me that this is a romantic thing we had going on. I just thought, "This is what girls do, we have super besties!" I saw our whole lives together as best friends, except that I would get a boyfriend at some point. And then in college, I told my first real girlfriend what we'd done and she was like, "Erika, best friends don't do that. Girlfriends do that."

Throughout my whole life, falling into relationships with women was so easy and effortless and intense. It didn't even occur to me that this could be an option for a romantic partner. I didn't know lesbians; this wasn't part of my concept for a relationship.

My mom is super homophobic. Even before I could acknowledge what my feelings were for girls, she would take me aside and physically pin me down or against a wall and say, "Tell me you're straight. Tell me you're straight." She wouldn't let me go until I'd told her I was straight.

So my feelings for girls: I wasn't in a place where I could acknowledge that this was a romantic feeling.

When I was like 17, I made internet friends with this righteous, feminist dyke. It was on the internet that I started to become comfortable with the bisexual label even though, personally, I didn't have any sexual experience in any regard. Then I went to college and this girl came around a corner and I felt like I'd been struck by lightning. That became the first person I ever had an adult relationship with.

I was so confused. I didn't know if I was just fascinated with this girl—I didn't know if I could be physical with her. I'd had penetrative sex once, with an internet boyfriend, and that was my only reference point. I thought, "Maybe I just really like her, maybe it's not sexual." Finally, we were hanging out talking and I said, "Hey, uh, I really want to kiss you." She leaned in and then I was like, "Wait! I don't remember how!" And she whispered, "I'll show you." So that was my first kiss with a girl. It was awesome! It was the best kiss I've ever had in my life! I was like, "Okay, I can do this physical thing."

I was crazy in love with her. We dated off and on for three years; she kept breaking up with me.

You can love someone, but that doesn't mean you are good for each other. You can love somebody, care about somebody, but that doesn't mean you're good together. I mean, I love peanuts. They're my favorite food. And I became allergic to them. It's the worst. Just because you love someone doesn't mean it's enough to sustain a relationship. Like, my mom loves me. And she's my mom, so there's a part of me that will always love her. But she is toxic; really bad for me. I cut her out of my life a few years ago. Love is not enough, if someone's hurting you.

My ex in college would dump me regularly because, well, to be fair, I was a basket case. I was in love for the first time and I've struggled with depression and anxiety my whole life—but she was also a dick. We loved each other! I know we're supposed to be talking about romantic relationships, but that's something I also learned from my mother, who is a certifiably crazy person.

Even if you love someone, you have to be good partners, to support each other. No one is perfect. To this day, I struggle with depression and anxiety, but we, Matt and me, we can communicate and support each other, we know how to express our feelings in a positive way. We never call each other names, not for real.

But back to my girlfriend and me. You can have two good people and put them together and it makes it toxic. My friends told me, "Erika, you can't keep doing this." It was so hard, because, like, being in love with her was like breathing air. I couldn't not do it.

Sexuality Can Be Too Complicated For Labels

I started college thinking I was bisexual. Then being with a woman and how fulfilling that was and how that worked sexually, I thought, "Oh! This is it! Those crushes I had on boys—I was lying to myself. I'm a dyke!" The thought of touching a man made me feel physically ill. And then when I was studying abroad in France, I went to England. And I met this British boy.

Matt had been a fan of my comics and when I was going to England, I wrote on my Livejournal, "Hey! I'm going to England! Anyone want to hang out?" I was 21; I would never do that today. Matt offered to let me stay at his place. I sent him an email saying, "I'm a lesbian, don't think you can try anything." And he was like, "No! It's okay!"

I don't believe in love at first sight. I don't think that's a thing. But when I saw the two people I've ever fallen in love with, my girlfriend and Matt, I had a full body electric shock.

All my lesbian friends back at college had all hooked up with guys at some point. I was like, "I'm going to hook up with this British boy and I'll have a great story to tell my friends back home." I thought it would be a once-in-a-lifetime thing. I spent all weekend hitting on him as hard as I could, just blatant. But he remembered that email I'd sent and was just like, "Well, American lesbians are so friendly." Finally, I was just like, "Hey, want to make out?" He was 19. He'd never had a girlfriend before.

I wasn't like, "This shall be a boyfriend." I was just like, "I like this guy." Matt and I kept in contact; we kept texting each other. On the spur of a moment, I invited him on a trip around France and on that trip, we fell in love.

When Going Long Distance, Invest In Phone Sex

For three-and-a-half-years, we had this long-distance relationship, from England to Portland. Long distance is not sustainable but we talked every day. All of my money went to buying phone cards, and his did too. I memorized the entire code—the card number, the pin, and the dialing England number. With the eight-hour time distance, he would ring me when it was time to get up in the morning. On my lunch break, I would call him and he would be in bed.

We didn't think, "We're going to be together someday." We always said, if I met someone here or he met someone in England, we would be like, "Go for it." We didn't think we had a future together. We were just like, "We're going to do this until we can't anymore." But going a day without talking to him was horrible.

The thing we learned is that you have to know when you're going to see each other again. It makes it hurt less. We figured out that we could afford to see each other every three months—we'd each pay for half a ticket each time.

Another key was phone sex. We had a lot of phone sex. It forced us to really talk about sex stuff and what we were into.

We thought we would date other people, but then there was no one else. I would get crushes on people, but Matt would be like, "Please, just don't flirt with them. Don't do that, because I'm not there, it's a threat to me when you feel like that for other people." There was some jealousy there, but now that we're together, it's cool when I get crushes on people; he encourages that.

It's Your Job To Speak Up

I don't believe that there's one person out there for you, like storybook love, that stuff you see in movies. And yet, I'm living it. I am happy every day when I wake up and see him there. It takes work, but it's not hard. I try to give Matt a positive reinforcement every day, tell him something I appreciate about him so that he knows I don't take him for granted. We're both people who are prone to being depressed and feeling lonely and knowing that you have this other person who does love you and you love them too, that goes a long way.

He is my other half—which you're probably not supposed to say if you're an independent feminist woman, but he's my partner. I struggle with that feeling, because he also earns a lot more money than I do. Could I be an independent lady if I didn't have Matt? I worry that I'm not pulling my weight. I also feel like: maybe my accomplishments don't count because what enables me to be a full-time cartoonist is the fact that I don't have to earn enough to support two people. But Matt wants my career to take off. If I was dicking around and not working hard, he would not be okay with it. But he sees that I work my ass off. So, no, it's not just "a wife's hobby." This is my career, I'm working at it seven days a week.

When you're in a relationship, you need to talk honestly. Don't be passive. Don't be passive aggressive. If you feel something, it is your job to speak up. You have to put it in words, like a grown up. Even with my high school bestie, she would do things that I didn't like—just as friends interacting—and I could not speak up and criticize her. I could not say, "I don't like it when you do this."

I think Matt is maybe the only person I can speak to directly about how I'm feeling about things. We have to talk about what we're feeling and not rely on subtle clues or expect him to read my mind or, if I'm upset, just go outside and sulk. If he does something that upsets me, I say, "Hey, buddy, when you did that thing, that was not cool." It's actually talking to someone, communicating—not doing passive aggressive bullshit.

Threesomes Can Be Terrifying

Ever since I became sexually active, I've always thought it was super hot to think that other people are attracted to my partner, to think that my partner could go off and fuck somebody. I've always been into that. It's titillating. I like my partners being independent sexual beings on their own; not in relation to me. However, I've never thought about opening up my own relationships. Then, several years ago, Matt was like, "Threesomes sound kind of hot." And I was like, "I like the idea, but in reality doesn't that tear apart relationships?" The jealousy! He was like, "Well, you know, let's take baby steps." So it was initially his idea.

We talked about what we wanted from a threesome buddy. We weren't just like, "Let's try it and see how it goes!" We wanted to figure out as much as we could ahead of time. How involved did we want this person to be in our lives? Who can be in the pool of options? How do you treat that person when they're with us? How do you talk about them when they're not there? Who has contact with that person? Matt and I came up with the "no friend" rule, because if you fuck a friend, you already care about that person. And then if you throw sex into that, things can get complicated.

Matt and I made a listing on an adult website looking for a third and got a bunch of emails back from people. We went through a website because we wanted it to be structured— we all know why we were there. You think it's something that just kind of happens, but instead, it takes a lot of planning.

We actually did have a threesome once before, with my original high school super bestie. She visited us and was being super flirty. It wasn't a good experience for Matt, he was so anxious. It took years before we talked about trying a threesome again.

I was surprised at how cool I was with it; I was not upset to see my high school friend and my boyfriend on each other. He got both of us off, but it was not a great experience for him.

Make Your Main Partnership Front And Center

After we signed up for the adult website, we went through the process of emailing back and forth with people, looked at their pictures, and finally met up with this guy—in a public place, of course.

I was so terrified. We had this initial awkward small talk like, "Ha ha! I like pumpkin pie! What kind of pie do you like?" And then he directed the conversation, saying, "So, why did you guys sign up for that website?" He was not somebody I would necessarily seek out as my partner, but he was nice and communicative. He asked the questions that we didn't know we should be asking. He asked about all sorts of boundaries, like what we would be interested in doing. We told him we're pretty vanilla and had a verbal disclosure of sexual health. But when we left, in my head, I was like, "Nope! Shut it down! Can't fuck a stranger!" Matt was like, "I think it could be alright." I was like, "Really?" and he was like, "Look at his body!" And so I agreed to go along with it just for the sake of doing it once. I was scared.

Then the threesome we had—it was freakin' awesome! I had such a good time! We had the ground rule that we wouldn't have penetrative sex. We just rolled around and played with each other's junk. It completely energized me. For days afterwards, I felt like I was on a high. For Matt, it was a bit like, "Oh geez, that was a little much for me." I was so jazzed by this whole experience that I kept saying to Matt, "Wasn't that great?! Can you believe when he blah blah blah?!" Then I realized that it wasn't just about me feeling elated. I had to be like, "Baby, you're my partner. I love you."

We've been seeing the same guy for about three years, three or four times a year. We call him our sex friend. We have threesomes when Matt feels comfortable.

We get along with our sex friend really well. He's not in our life at all, except for being our fuck-buddy every few months. We treat our sex friend well; we hang out with him afterwards. Our special guest star comes in and we have a great time and it spices things up. But it's clear that this is the Matt and Erika show.

Do What Feels Sexy To You

I travel a lot and Matt has been like, "Hey, if you find someone you want to fuck on your trip, you can go for it." He'll pack little condoms in my suitcase. I almost took him up on that on this one trip, but I chickened out at this last minute—I probably made this guy think I'm a total tease. I came back and I told Matt all about it. I recounted the whole story and he pounced on me—in a good, consensual way, of course. Then we've used that story for role-playing stuff. This outside element helps us have fun sex and keep it interesting, even though 99 percent of the time, we are the ones who are just fucking each other.

I've been giving him permission to sleep with other people way longer than he's been giving me permission. Whenever I go out of town, I've been like, "Honey, there's some things I can't do very well. You have total permission to do that stuff with someone else." The idea of him sleeping with someone else is totally hot to me. If someone else gets to sleep with Matt, I'd be like, "Yeah! He's a good lay!" I'm sure I'd have some jealously but, conceptually, I think that's fine, as long as we tell each other. If you sleep with someone else, you're still coming back to me at the end. You love me, but you get to be this hot piece of ass. I love the idea of other people looking at him, hitting on him, wanting to sleep with him. It's not fair that I'm the only person who gets to sleep with him. It feels like hoarding.

4.

Gender
is
Messy

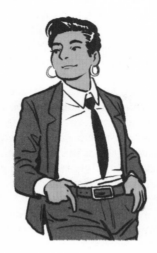

Even kids know that gender isn't simple.

We're taught when we're young that boys only do boy-things and think in boy-ways and girls only do girl-things and think in girl-ways. But for as long as I can remember, those rules rubbed me the wrong way. As a kid, I felt like a girl, but I thought it was silly to act only in girl-ways. I liked being both girly *and* a tomboy. I liked to wear dresses *and* I liked to roughhouse. I often played with the dolls *and* I never crossed my legs. I didn't want to be a princess, but I didn't want to be a prince, either. My role models were girls who went outside the roles of their gender, women who were a little "weird": Pippi Longstocking, Laura Ingalls Wilder, Harriet the Spy.

We spend our lives mixing and matching, learning to craft our identities for ourselves—and, often, wishing that being who we want to be involved less hassle, less unlearning, and fewer dismissive encounters. I'm a woman and I've always identified as a woman, but *performing* my gender has often been tricky: I rarely want to behave the way women are supposed to behave—but when my desired behaviors do line up with the norm, I resent myself for being so traditional. I feel good about myself and my body these days, but I frequently wish gender were easier.

That feeling of confusion and insecurity about how I'm supposed to be a woman becomes especially acute while dating. When I'm going on a date with a new guy, I worry over whether I should be more feminine—I've always wanted to be one of those girls who smells nice and has the perfect shoes and I know that's never going to happen. In long-term relationships, the problems get deeper as I start to recognize how expectations around gender affect my behavior and my partner's behavior in big ways. A major part of learning how I want to act in relationships has involved realizing that those childhood set-in-stone gender rules are actually very fluid. What an exciting discovery!

An invaluable resource for me as I think about my gender has been conversations with transgender friends. To get to the point where they can identify with a gender their parents' didn't expect, or with no gender at all, each of my transgender friends had to do some deep thinking. They've had to examine big, scary ideas of sexuality and gender roles and learned how they want to build their own unique identity.

Our conversations make me realize how gender rules are just stories I've been told over and over again. Not coming into conflict with those stories has been a privilege for me in many ways. For all my frustrations over how society expects women to be pretty and polite, every day I take for granted the dozens of ways that I conform to other peoples' expectations of how a woman should behave, including how I look, what I wear, my demeanor, and the sound of my voice. Many transgender folks tell me that they can't *not* think about gender roles every day. Since they're chafing at some of the basic assumptions of our culture, they perceive rules, expectations, and problems that fly right past me.

Since the perspectives in this chapter are coming from people who have thought a lot about gender and sexuality with a critical eye, this is good relationship advice for all types of people. Everyone can benefit from thinking more critically about gender—these conversations have helped me feel more comfortable with wearing "feminine" outfits *and* with acting in assertive "masculine" ways. In part because of our conversations, I feel better about acting how I genuinely want to.

The Details

Our society is pretty rigid about gender. We've got two: girls and boys. But what it means to be a girl or boy is an elaborate idea we've built up over generations. Many people feel uneasy with this idea and the partition of people into one camp or the other.

Instead of seeing gender as a distinct either-or choice, some people see gender as a spectrum: some people definitely feel like women, some people definitely feel like men, some people feel like both ideas are not quite right and they're a gender somewhere in the middle. Some people reject the whole concept of being male or female as socially constructed hogwash.

We also link gender with sex. If someone is born with female genitalia, we assume they'll grow up to be a woman. If someone is born with male genitalia, we assume they'll grow up to be a man. But lots of people are assigned a gender at birth, based on their genitalia, and then come to understand later on that they don't identify as that gender at all. Though they're born with female genitalia, for example, they've always felt like they're a man. Or they're born with a penis, but have felt like they're not a man or a woman—no label feels right. In other cases, people are born with genitalia that's not clearly male or female so a doctor makes the call on what their gender assignment should be.

For most people, gender never fits quite right. For some people, the annoyance is mild like mine. For other people, the disruptive feeling runs much deeper.

These days, the term "transgender" is used to describe all sorts of people whose birth-assigned sex and their own internal sense of their gender do not match. There are different identities that fit under the term transgender, including people who want to get sex reassignment surgery to match their gender identity, people who don't want surgery, and people who are in the process of taking hormones or considering surgery. The terms genderqueer and agender are used to describe people who feel like they're not comfortable being considered male or female. There are so many different ways to identify if you're transgender that people use the word trans* to stand in for all the diverse identities that can loosely be called transgender. One tricky language issue with *not* identifying as either male or female is that you need pronouns that don't label you as male or female. Some examples of gender-neutral pronouns are *ze*, *xe*, or just *they* instead of he or she.

I'm what's called cisgender, by the way. The prefix "trans" means "to cross over" while "cis" means "same side." So that means my assigned gender at birth matches my gender identity today: Though I resent a lot of the behaviors that people expect of women, I still feel like a woman.

When talking about how the male/female gender is a specific idea that we've created, it's useful to look at how cultures recognized gender throughout history. In America, we only have two legally recognized genders. But other countries and cultures have more genders. Numerous native cultures, like the Mohave, Zuni, Lakota, and Zapotec people in North America had words for third genders. Words for third-gendered people have also been documented in India and Thailand. The first set of laws written down in human history, the Code of Hammurabi, made note of third-gender people who were born female but had male traits.

10 Lessons From Trans* Folks
1. Gender weighs heavy on everyone.

Think about what we consider masculine and feminine. It's silly, when you break it down. The way people dress, the way they part their hair, and the way they walk down the street all play into our perceptions of whether they're male or female. We're using these clues all the time to hold up the ideas ingrained in us. When we start to screw around with those ideas, it can be fun and feel more genuine. Going against those ideas is tough. It's work! It can make you feel sad and crazy! It's like a job, only you don't get paid. You just get to wear cute stuff. "If I'd been comfortable trying to live as a man, I probably would," says Berkeley activist Root, who was born male and now identifies as genderqueer. "It's definitely the path of least resistance. But masculinity was this exhausting burden I had to bear."

2. **Listen to your friends.**

   Gender is tough, right? So when friends or dates *do* speak up about how they feel, how they're worried about being seen, and how they want to be seen—it's your job to listen and take their words to heart. One major thing that people who are trans* deal with is people not taking them seriously, like saying they're faking it or it's just a phase. Peoples' relationship to their gender does change throughout their life and it's our job as kind and respectful humans to understand the work it takes to sort through all that stuff. Speaking up about feeling different requires incredible trust—so honor that. Support your friends where they're at and behave toward them in the way they ask you to. People who are trans* sometimes change their names and gender identities and it can take time for their friends to adapt. It's understandable that it takes time to adapt to a new identity, as long as you're sincere and respectful along the way.

3. **Don't put people on the spot about their gender.**

   Everyone has parts of their identity they like to keep private and it's not your right to know those most private parts of someone. For example, it wouldn't be appropriate to walk up to someone who looks like a woman and ask about her vagina. You wouldn't ask her how she feels about being a woman. Don't ask the same questions of people who are trans* or seem genderqueer. Inquiring whether they're "really" a man or are going to get surgery is rude. If you sincerely want to know how they feel about their identity, take the time and energy to build a relationship that's deep and safe enough that you both feel comfortable talking about gender. If you're not up for that, you're not up for a friendship—you have the kind of questions Google can answer.

4. **But do talk about gender.**

   Pestering someone about their genitalia is not the same as having genuine, vulnerable conversations about gender with people you know well. That kind of conversation is great! As some gender theory folks say, "All gender is drag." It can be really nice to hash out with friends why we act the way we do. Think about how and why you identify the way you do and how you express that. Then, with your good friends and people you're dating, explain the ways you identify. When Root and ze's college girlfriend talked about gender identity, for example, she was able to bring up the ways she felt judged for being traditionally feminine—she liked to sew, she liked cooking, she liked wearing poofy dresses.

5. **Your parents aren't always going to get it.**

This goes for partners, too. But there's a difference between bigoted people who don't care about you and people who genuinely care about you and have trouble understanding the ways that you're dealing with gender. It's understandable that people react strongly if you seem to change—they care about you and want you to be happy. Boston resident Leila was born female but identifies now as genderqueer. Leila's parents still want to think of Leila as their "daughter" and with female pronouns—Leila's not into that, but understands that it will take them a long time to wrap their minds around an identity that's different than they expected. If you start to act in ways that are against gender norms, even in the tiniest of ways, people are going to give you the side-eye. My mom still reminds me that there's a razor in the shower when I haven't shaved my legs for a few months. Other peoples' parents and partners start to notice when they begin acting in a more masculine or more feminine way, like changing their style or their hair. Try to help them understand by opening up to them about what makes you happy and what makes you sad.

6. **Find a community that understands you.**

This is the most important point of all. Wherever you land on the gender spectrum, you're not alone. You've got to somehow find people you can talk to about how you feel and what you want. Whether it's friends, family, or communities online; as you grapple with gender, it helps to know that other people are thinking about the same issues. Recognizing that you're not the way our culture expects you to be can feel alienating. You've got to find allies. Some people think of this as making their own family. Even if you're not changing gender identity, you need a community that doesn't alienate you because of how you identify.

7. **Date people who care about you.**

   This is part of building a community. Date people who are a support, not people who make you feel uncomfortable. Finding a supportive partner can be a great part of exploring gender.

8. **Respect your partners' pace.**

   We're taught the golden rule: "Do unto others as you want done unto you." Consider this modification: Do unto others as they want done. Meaning, just because you're comfortable doesn't mean the other person is comfortable. Getting physically intimate with partners can bring up all kinds of scary issues around gender and bodies. Give the people you care about space to express themselves and take time to listen and process what they're saying. It'll help you understand more about yourself too.

9. **Recognize your own privilege.**

   Our thoughts on how dating is supposed to work and how people are supposed to act are based a lot on our personal backgrounds. It comes from race, class, gender identity, and sexual orientation. It comes from history. An essential part of understanding why we think the way we do comes from recognizing the privileges we have: what do we take for granted? What do we assume other people want and need and how do they identify? How do those ideas play into how we date people? These are the kinds of questions it takes a lifetime to unpack but, hey! That's our responsibility. Let's get on it.

10. **Create a comfortable identity.**

    We create our own identities from different stories we like. If you want to wear skirts, wear skirts. If you want to wear combat boots and bow ties, more power to you. Once you recognize that gender is silly, it's worth playing with. Portlander Ledah, who is genderqueer, wrote a letter to their 88-year old grandma about their identity. "My grandma immediately called me and said, 'Do whatever you need to do to be happy,'" says Ledah, "It's so rare. It's really sweet. It's like, you just want me to be happy as a human. She's the best person I know."

Last Thoughts

Recently, a very professional eighth grader interviewed me for a documentary she was making about body image. This was her first documentary, but she assured me, definitely not her last. We sat in my office for a long time while she asked me big questions and recorded me on her camera phone. I talked about how gender can feel like a box that very few people fit neatly into.

"Why is it a box?" she asked.

That question stopped me—I use the "gender is a box" metaphor so often that I hadn't really thought it about it deeply.

"It works two ways," I answered, after a long pause. One way is that there's a circumscribed set of behaviors and rules about gender and if we venture outside of that narrow area, we face stigma. In that way, gender norms are a box that we have to stay inside of to be safe. The other way to think about gender is as a checklist, a series of boxes that we're supposed to tick off to fit in perfectly. Getting intimate with someone can make that checklist seem more real and dire—as I size myself up in someone else's eyes, I become acutely aware of how I'm not the "ideal" girl. The young filmmaker knew just what I was talking about. My anxiety over ways I'm weird had reached a fever pitch during eighth grade but has been reliably ebbing since then.

In my best romantic relationships, when I'm alone with the person I'm dating, the checklist seems to dissolves into irrelevance. It's been valuable.

STU RASMUSSEN

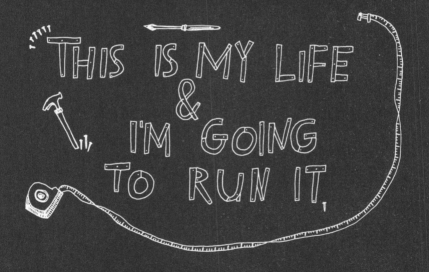

"THIS IS MY LIFE & I'M GOING TO RUN IT"

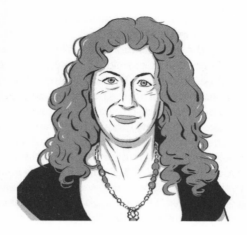

Stu Rasmussen is a great small-town mayor. A frank and funny native of Silverton, Oregon, Stu runs the town movie theater on Main Street, is an local enthusiastic business booster, and has a lot of strong opinions about smart economic policies. But when the rural town elected him in 2008, the local politician made headlines nationwide. Stu is America's first transgender mayor—he was born a man, but is now (he'll gladly tell you) the proud bearer of 36DD breasts, an extensive dress collection, and identifies as neither a man nor a woman. You'll often find him in the afternoon outside of his theater, standing on the street corner in heels to greet neighbors, talk politics, and maybe even sell some movie tickets.

I talked with Stu in the office of the downtown copy center run by his wife Victoria, who occasionally chimed in with a snide comment.

Ease Into Change

I had a very slow transition over 30 or 40 years.

I wish I could point to something in my past that said, "Aha! That was the seminal moment where I realized I was transgender." But I didn't even know the word transgender until about fifteen years ago. I grew up here and it's a small town, I didn't have a lot of access to information. You would hear stories about male to female transitions, but only as magazine freakshow. I knew I was different around puberty, which was when I started crossdressing. I enjoyed looking like a female; I enjoyed looking in the mirror and seeing a female me look back at me. Why, how? I have no idea.

Not everybody is short, not everybody is tall—we're somewhere in between. I think I'm 40 to 50 percent between male and female. I do a lot of male things, I do a lot of female things. It's not a binary system; there are shades of gray.

When I moved to Portland [in 1968], I had a little more freedom to express my gender variance, but I was closeted for years. I would wear women's clothing in the closet, but never go out, not even fantasize about it. Or, a couple times, I'd be afraid to go out in the daylight so I'd go out at night. Which, come to think of it, is the most dangerous behavior you could do. I don't know that I ever encountered another cross-dresser, I don't know where I would have gone to do so.

My awakening came with the internet in the late 80s. Anonymously poking around on there, I found that I was not all that unusual. There's a big world out there of people who are differently gendered. I slowly crawled out of my shell. At that time, there weren't websites, just bulletin boards where you could post a message and other people could respond. I was up all hours of the night reading them. I was not alone.

That led me to find a Portland transgender social and support group in the early 90s called the Northwest Gender Alliance. I called an anonymous phone number and stammered to this voice on the end and they invited me to the meeting. I thought I was going to a freakshow. I went in boy clothes, as most people do the first time out, because you're just not comfortable cross-dressing in public. And it was weird; these guys were perfectly smart and normal except for this little piccadilly of liking to dress as women.

I talked to airline pilots, engineers, school teachers, marine architects, and truck drivers; we just shared this quirk. For some, it was a stop on the road toward a sex change. For others, it was all that they wanted, the opportunity to express themselves in the opposite gender. I thought that's where I was for a long time, until the allure of cleavage came up.

Find Partners Who Have Got Your Back

In the seventies, I got a job working for a movie theater chain in Portland. In the 5th Avenue Cinema, there was a lovely young thing there selling tickets and popcorn. She was still in high school when we met, but I was smitten. Horribly. I'll never get over it. We communicate mostly by grunts and sign language, these days. We're very similar people, it's a continuous source of annoyance.

If you're just getting started in a relationship these days, I would go for 80 percent candor. A relationship that's been going for a while, five years, ten years, it's almost dishonest to bring it out then, but you have to do it.

I was conflicted over the cross-dressing, but I was not conflicted in my own mind over whether I was heterosexual. The male hormones had taken over and I was on the prowl. I wasn't comfortable cross-dressing in front of Victoria, but I finally came out to her about six years into our relationship. This monumental angst had been building up in me through the whole relationship. Eventually I was like, "Honey, there's this thing that I have to do." And her response was, "Meh, okay." It was kind of an anticlimax.

Victoria: If my mother had warned me about men like you, it might have been different. But she didn't and it just didn't seem like that big of a deal to me. I mean, I'd been wearing slacks for as long as I could. If you'd been thinking about [vaginal construction] surgery, I think it would have been different. I wasn't getting into this to live with another woman, so that would be a big deal for me.

We didn't equate gender with sexuality, we both understood we were heterosexual. I was not leaving Victoria for another man or woman.

I think a large part of our relationship dynamic is still male-female. Even though I happen to look like a woman sometimes, we're still very conventional. Perhaps too conventional. She makes dinner every night. She's a good cook.

When I decided I wanted breasts, Victoria and I had a couple discussions about it. I said, "What I'd really like is breasts, how would you feel about that?" It was not a big deal, as far as I can tell. We had a lot of issues in the relationship, but the gender issue just wasn't one of them. I think that's 99 percent thanks to Victoria.

There was a lot of talk in town before that, a lot of buzzing because I'd been easing into the transition, wearing bright red nails sometimes. I think Victoria took the worst of it, people asking, "What's up with Stu and the nails?" She'd day, "Why don't you ask Stu?"

You Need A Community—Whatever That Looks Like

Some of the trans people I knew had moved to Portland from podunk, where they had a life that couldn't express their gender identity and they thought that moving to the big city and starting over again would be the panacea to make it work. And for some, I think they were right.

If your family isn't supportive, if you grew up in a family with strict gender roles assigned, it would be very difficult to come out. But if you move, you're uprooting yourself from everything that you know and love and starting over again in a place where you don't know anybody or anything and you're trying to do it all in a new body. That's a very steep hill to climb.

For me, it was such a slow transition that everybody in Silverton just kind of came along with it. So it worked for me, but I don't know if it would work for everyone. If I could do it all over again, would I do the tempting thing and move to a big city and start over there? No, absolutely not. Victoria and I moved back to Silverton in the mid-80s. I was a closeted cross-dresser but outwardly as macho as this little guy could get. I ran the town movie theater and the TV channel, so I kept that other part of my personality submerged.

I first ran for city council in 1984 and served for about ten years, but after I was no longer on the council, that's when I was reading a lot online started thinking about what I wanted to do and what would make me happy. I was done with politics as far as I knew, so I thought I would do what I wanted.

On March 1, 2000, the twins came into the world. I did not dress much as a woman before the breast augmentation. Even after that, it was about a year of working up to dressing around town in the full regalia. It was something that was hard for me, but I took baby steps. I pushed the community a little bit, they pushed back a little bit, until finally it was just, "Oh that's just Stu. He's a little weird, but he's a halfway decent guy...a halfway decent girl. Halfway decent whatever."

In retrospect, I think 99 percent of what I was afraid of was between my ears, that I wasn't ready or that I was uncertain of myself. I wish I knew what I was scared of. Public reaction, I guess. I was concerned about how the community would support my business with a freakshow owning it. Business did drop, but it came back.

In 2004, people were pretty much used to me in town, I ran for city council again, and I'm sure behind my back there was a lot of hubbub, but I made a good case and got elected. I think it's a small enough town that most people know me— good or bad. I have a reputation for an abiding care for the community. It's genuine, it's not a political statement; my heart is here. This is the community I grew up in, so there's just no question about that.

I think we're at the point where people overlook my appearance and vote for me as a person. It's clearly not a beauty contest around here, because then I'd be in deep doo-doo.

Stupidity Hurts
I don't mind any pronoun other than "it."

To people around town who've gotten used to me as Stu over the past 60 years, I'm still a "he." People who got to know me in other lifestyles know me as "she." It doesn't really matter to me, I don't care which pronoun they use. That's one of the problems with gender presentation, the first time people meet you, they don't know what pronoun to use and they don't want to offend you—or they do want to offend you—and they stumble over it. It's really hard for someone who's not in the transgender community to know what pronoun to use and not be offensive.

If you just get past that and don't care, your life smoothes out. It's still amusing to meet someone new and they think I'm female and they use female pronouns. When that happens, I think, "Oh good, I'm passing really well today." Or, "'Hey, you need to get glasses immediately."

Being in politics, you get a totally different feel for how this works. Half the people despise you even if you do the job well. So you just have to get over it.

I unseated the guy who'd been mayor for sixteen years and thought he was anointed rather than elected. He still has his cadre of darklings who find criticism with anything I do. I think my gender expression has a bit to do with that, and also that when I was elected and the news went worldwide, they were pissed as hell. Not only did their guy not win, but Silverton went in the spotlight because the people had dared to elect someone not of their mold as mayor.

But the people that hate me are a small percentage and they're easily ignored. It isn't relevant to my life what your opinion is because I know you're wrong. You may be under the impression that the sun rises in the north and sets in the south, but the facts are otherwise. It still hurts when you're dealing with stupid, and unfortunately there's no shortage of that.

At a younger age, I was concerned about others' opinions about me. I didn't want to do anything off the map. If my twenty-year-old self were in 2012, I'd say, "Buck up kid, just go do it." But talking to my twenty-year-old self in 1968, when the world didn't know anything about that, I would consider that advice insane. The position that I've put myself in has brought a lot of young people to me, asking for advice and I tell them, "You have to be true to yourself and go do it."

Gender identity is none of your damn business; get over it. Once you realize: this is my life and I'm going to run it, things become a lot easier.

5.

Staying Childless By Choice

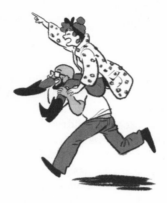

....

I'll be honest: I don't like kids. The smaller, the scarier, I say.

I'm the younger sister in my four-person family, so I didn't grow up with babies as a part of my daily life. These days, I live in a city where my days are full of work and movies and bars and bike rides. Babies are a rare and distant part of other peoples' lives, not mine. They seem like foreign, squishy, fragile objects.

So it's hard to wrap my brain around the idea that I'm actually capable of making a real, live baby—much less that I would desire to raise one so badly that I would give my life over to it. Every movie ever made tells me that my biological clock will kick in someday soon; a mothering instinct will ambush my apathy. But so far, no dice.

Having a baby will be my choice, but not one I'll make alone. This issue will someday be a major part of my relationships. And being undecided on the baby question leaves me vulnerable to being talked into a life that I don't want. Worst case scenario would be one day looking down into my baby's tiny, beady eyes for the first time and finally realizing what I want: Whoops! I was never meant to be a mother. I need to figure out what I actually want, stat.

Sure, having a baby is normal, but is it necessary? I have a lot I want to get done in my life and a lot of adventures I have yet to go on. My mom took five years off from her career to see my brother and I through toddler-hood, working nights at Macy's while she and my dad occasionally pawned possessions to buy diapers. Hearing of sacrifices like these makes me say a secret prayer to the birth control coursing through my veins. Will I really someday want to reorient my life around having children? On the other hand, every child-bearing adult I know (my loving parents included) speaks sincerely about their kids being one of the most important parts of their lives. Clearly, children bring profound joy to many people. What deep, basic human experiences will I miss if I opt-out of utilizing my uterus?

The most important choice we make in life, it seems to me, is whether or not to have a baby. Yet for my whole life, I've only heard from the pro-baby camp. Speaking out against bearing children is impolite. Expressing regret over having kids is entirely taboo. Since instinct is clearly not guiding me on whether or not to have a kid, I think the only way to make an honest, informed decision about whether to have kids, is to balance out our culture's constant pro-baby propaganda and talk to people who've decided to never have children.

The Details
Modern technology has overcome ancient biology, so now sexually active people are in a luxurious situation: they are able to decide for themselves whether or not to procreate.

People who spend their lives childless by choice aren't just expressing practical concerns around overpopulation and the costs of childbearing. Aiming to never have kids challenges the concept of what makes a family. Dating and marriage are traditionally viewed as merely a path to the ultimate expression of "true love": having a child together. People who are childless by choice redefine their romantic and sexual relationships as being about the relationship itself, not being any sort of vehicle for procreation.

So how much of an oddball would I be, really, if I decide to never have kids? Well, the 2010 Census revealed that having a child is less and less a requirement for being a mainstream American family: There are now more American homes with dogs than children. Across the country, women are having fewer kids and having them later. It's no longer that weird to be a mom in your forties, and it's also becoming increasingly less weird to not be a mom at all. In 2010, a little more than eight percent of middle-aged Americans said they expected to have no children, a significant jump from the 1970s.

So every childless person chooses to not have kids for their own reasons, but researchers over the past few decades have found some things in common among the group. People who are childfree are more likely to live in cities, less likely to be religious, more likely to have graduated from college, and more likely to be financially stable than their child-bearing peers. Childfree people don't have to deal with years of diapers and angsty teens, but choosing not to have kids is laden with its own challenges: Childfree people will likely face stigma from their peers and flack from their family.

However, don't let neighbors' whispers or your grandma's sighs goad you into having children if you think being a parent might not be the right choice for you. A child should be a conscious choice, not an accident or an obligation. The people interviewed for this chapter all made the tough choice to be sterilized or use long-term birth control and they're all happy with the relationships they've built for themselves without kids in the picture.

Fifteen Lessons From People Who Are Childless By Choice

1. Accept that, for some people, "mothering instinct" is a myth.

As women get into their late twenties, thirties, and forties, they keep thinking that some switch will flip and suddenly they'll want kids. But for whatever reason, it's clear that many women never find themselves desiring kids. Figuring that out has meant sitting themselves down and considering how kids have affected the lives of friends and family.

Vivian is a Portlander in her late twenties, a graphic designer and bike racer. While it seems like all her friends are getting married and popping out children, her fiancé just got a vasectomy. "Seeing my friends having kids has forced me to really think, 'This is just not for me.' It hasn't ever been a conscious choice. I just knew that having kids was not something I was interested in."

But I'm not alone in having no clear instinct about babies. Many people expressed that they have never been 100 percent sure if having kids is the right choice or not. Feelings change, lives change; there's no fertility lightning bolt that shoots down from the sky one day and strikes you, filling you with the Heaven-sent knowledge that you must be a parent. Instead, coming to terms with never having kids is more gradual and involves a lot of talking things out honestly with friends or partners. At some point, though, biology forces you to take the plunge one way or another.

2. **Talk about babies—they're a deal breaker.**

Everyone agrees: Children are not the kind of relationship issue on which you and a partner can meet halfway, other than, perhaps, fostering a child for a limited number of years. You can't make half a baby, or just agree to have a tiny child of your own. That means you have to have actual, honest conversations with long-term partners about whether you want kids. But seeing as how half of pregnancies are unintentional, it seems like a lot of people are skipping or evading this crucial conversation.

"If you're dating, you need to figure out whether or not you want children so you can be open about it from the first time you meet someone. It's a deal breaker," says Ellen, who often talks about child-rearing issues in her therapy practice. "If you're already in a relationship, you do have to sit down together and figure it out and not just let fate decide."

That doesn't mean jumping to the baby conversation with new or casual partners (baby talk is not super effective first-date pillow talk). But figuring out whether you want kids and then discussing the issue in-depth should definitely happen before big commitments, like moving in together or getting married.

Some people rehash the idea of kids over and over with partners, some people do a lot of soul-searching on their own and find themselves on the same page as their partners. Art teacher Ally, 32, was a waffler. So was her partner Bruce. "I feel like we talked about it every day for a year," says Ally. "We go back and forth a bit, sometimes liking the idea. But at the end of the day, the answer is no."

Vivian, the twenty-something Portlander, was nervous to bring up her desire to never have kids with her partners. She was glad when her now-fiancé brought up the issue of kids after they'd been dating for about six months and were talking about where their relationship was going. "We were formulating whether we'd be compatible long term," says Vivian. "He was really explicit about it: He thought kids were expensive and a burden. I felt so relieved."

Not talking honestly with partners about whether you want kids is only going to end badly. Breaking up or getting divorced over not wanting kids is far better than bringing a human into the world who will receive less love and support than they deserve.

3. **We really don't need more humans in the world.**

On top of work and instinct, many people believe that not having kids is an ethical choice, given overpopulation and our penchant for monstrous consumption of resources. Environmental concerns are rarely the number one reason people have for not having kids, but it certainly backs up the choice and makes people feel like their against-the-norm decision is a just one.

The fact of the matter is that we're not going to be running out of humans any time soon. And we're a messy bunch: The average American creates over four pounds of garbage a day (even after they're out of diapers). Many people believe that not reproducing fits within their ethics of trying to reduce their environmental impact and not contribute to the overpopulation crisis. These issues weigh more heavily on people who came of age in the past twenty years, more so than they've weighed on any previous generation. After being taught all our lives to reduce, reuse, and recycle, the desire to be moral citizens of the earth tip the baby scales to "no" for some people who are deeply uncertain about whether having kids is the right thing to do with their lives.

The only person I talked to who put environmental concerns at the top of his list of reasons not to reproduce is Lint, a 33-year-old who works six months of the year in a warehouse to pay for spending the rest of the year as an avid long-distance backpacker. A tattoo on his upper thigh sums up his ideals: It's a baby crossed out, encircled by the words, "Fewer people, more wilderness."

"I don't care how many cloth diapers you use or how many Priuses you buy, having a kid is still a huge carbon footprint," says Lint.

4. Children are extremely expensive.

How much is a life worth? Not to be crass, but it's about $12,500 a year—that's the average cost of raising a child in America, working out to a quarter million dollars by the time the little miracle turns 18. People without kids have significantly more disposable income at hand, which can mean more opportunities to pursue dreams.

Hanna is a twenty-something freelance writer living in Seattle with her long-term boyfriend. She is acutely aware that she wouldn't be able to live in her "ridiculous single-person apartment," working for freelance wages if she had kids. If Hanna decided to have kids, she would first need to build up a stockpile of money, then take a long time off from work, and then make her children a priority over the erratic lifestyle of a marginally paid writer. Just coming up with the money to create a stable, supportive home for a child would mean switching careers, since her paycheck varies wildly from month to month. As is, she can write around the clock for meager pay and still have the energy to volunteer around Seattle and babysit for her siblings.

"It's always seemed to me like there's only two paths: You can have a career, or you can have children," says Hanna. "I'm the first person in my family to graduate from college, and no one else did because they had children. I decided pretty early on that I'd rather have a very fulfilling and aggressive career rather than children."

5. People without kids can be more mobile and adventurous.

Being childless allows people to live lives that aren't rooted in one place. Lots of people who don't have kids are the type of people who often go on long trips and adventures, whether it's taking six months to hike the Pacific Crest Trail or deciding all of a sudden to move to Argentina. Rick, a middle-aged programmer, has spent his adult life moving between cities and spending lots of time traveling to big festivals; essentially traveling wherever the wind and his relationships take him.

"So much of what I've done with my life is about not being in one place for a long time," says Rick. A kid doesn't fit into that image.

Ellen is a 51-year-old therapist in Washington who revels in her ability to travel whenever she wants. "I think a lot of moms my age look at my life and think it's strange. They see all of the freedom that I have, the freedom of my time," she says.

6. Raising kids doesn't have to be your life's work.

In addition to instinct, a major factor in peoples' decision to not have children is their career. Raising kids is a full-time job and a passion. Many people have weighed the commitment and decided they would rather throw their time and energy into their life's work.

For women especially, the time frame for having kids can conflict with professional goals like going to grad school. Since becoming, say, a neurosurgeon can take ten years, women either have to schedule their pregnancies around their graduations, do double-duty as mothers and students, or cross their fingers that they'll remain fertile into their late thirties.

For some people, the thought of people who opt for work over children conjures up the image of an icy, manhating CEO woman and her male counterpart: a ruthless executive with a giant, lonely mansion. I'm sure those people exist somewhere outside of Ayn Rand novels, but the reality among work-minded people I interviewed is very different.

For Ellen, getting a PhD was number one on her life to-do list. "I got really busy with my life. I realized when

I was 45 that if I really wanted a child, I better get with it immediately. I did some soul searching and finalized my decision."

For everyone I talked to, for whom work was a big factor in their decision not to have kids, was extremely busy, but not wealthy. Instead, these are often people who throw themselves into volunteering with social causes and community projects as well as working hard at ambitious paying gigs. I relate to the sentiment. There are plenty of worthy causes in the world that could use my time and energy—in some ways, it's selfish to devote myself to raising kids instead of channeling more of my life toward social justice work.

In a similar way, Ally and her husband Bruce—who waffled over having kids—know that if they have kids, it will mean giving up money, time, and energy that they would rather use to work on their art.

"I know there are people who have kids and still find time to create, but I also see people who have kids and stop creating, or stop creating for a decade. There's nothing in my life that's as important to me as my creative life," says Ally, who logs countless unpaid hours as an educator with an arts and media nonprofit.

7. **Not having kids doesn't mean you hate kids.**

Just because you don't birth your own doesn't mean you'll have a life devoid of kids. Many people without children find joy from working with kids, helping friends and family with their own children, or investing more energy into their adult relationships and living on their own terms.

"I work with kids. I think I'm helping future generations by being a teacher," says Ally. "We basically decided that our art would be our children and that our relationship would be our primary relationship."

One assumption made about people—especially women—who don't want kids is that they had a terrible childhood. While almost every childless-by-choice person I talked to said they had a happy childhood and they came to a point of clarity about not having children by evaluating the positive aspects of their lives without kids, a few people did point to their own rocky upbringings as a major factor in their eventual decision. A couple people remember family resources being spread too thin between too many kids. Others have a strained relationship in their family and would rather build a "chosen family" than continue their own genetic line. For some people, sadly, blood relatives have created deep frustration and anger. Their gut instinct leads them to make a clean break and not have a baby who would someday be owed the chance to meet their family.

8. **You will be judged for not being a parent.**
   Some words used to describe perceptions of childless parents in studies of stigma: selfish, materialistic, less nurturing, less desirable.

   Ouch.

   It's disappointing that our society often views people without kids as abnormal outsiders. But, for now, that's the way it is: Americans equate parenthood with selflessness, normalcy, and safety. Many people with children see them as the best part of their lives and can look askance at folks who decide not to raise kids. For signs of stigma against non-parents, just close your eyes and imagine getting a political candidate ad in the mail. What's on that glossy postcard? Likely, the image of an aspiring politician posing in a power suit with his wife and children (and a dog would be good, too). People—especially women—who don't have kids often get the message: "You have failed as a human being because you failed to procreate." Or, at the very least, there's something wrong with you.

   When you think about it logically, the idea that someone is selfish for not wanting to have kids is absurd—it's not like the species appears to be dying off any time soon. Not creating an *unwanted* child is really rather thoughtful. But the stigma persists, as people without kids face frequent barbs about not being willing to put a kid's life before their own. You'll be called to account for your decision over and over, while people with kids are uniformly congratulated. It can feel deeply unfair.

   Children are the only part of your personal sex life that people feel free to interrogate you about on a regular basis. Grandparents and grocery clerks won't ask you questions like: "Do you like having sex with your boyfriend? How often do you do it?" but it's perfectly normal for them to inquire about whether you intend to get pregnant and then express their opinion on the matter. Children are a very present part of our lives; it is somewhat obvious who has them and who doesn't. For this reason, choosing not to have children is both a deeply personal choice and a very public one. Many people assume that everyone desires to someday have kids—going against the grain requires childless folks to often explain themselves and their reasoning.

9. **Parents often take the "no baby, ever" news hard.** It can seem like everyone has an opinion on your fertility—especially your parents. People who are childless by choice have found that the best way to talk with their family about their plans is to be direct, firm, and to clearly explain the rationale behind their decision. In their experience, some parents feel like their kids' decision not to have children is a harsh judgment of their own parenting. Even then, it's smart to recognize, appreciate, and be sensitive toward the genuine pain that some friends and relatives will feel as they come to terms with a future that is not full of your kids.

"I told her straight, 'Mom, I'm never going to give you a grandchild,'" says Ally. As a part of the queer community, Ally found most of her friends were supportive of her choice not to have kids—except for her best friend from growing up. "She says it's my duty to have a child, because she thinks I'm such an awesome person. But I tell her there are tons of awesome people who have not-so-great children. There's no guarantee who your kid is going to be."

The issue has created more family strain for Vivian, who is Chinese-American and an only child. "There's this really deep thinking in Chinese culture that you owe your life to your parents. It was understood that I would grow up and meet a nice guy, get married, and have a kid or two," says Vivian. When her fiancé got a vasectomy, Vivian waited to tell her parents, but then mentioned it to her mother one day on the phone, bringing up the issue suddenly like she does with all big news. But, says Vivian, her parents did not seem to really believe that she will *never* have kids. "Even now, when I talk casually with my mom, she doesn't seem to acknowledge that it's a reality."

10. But don't assume your family won't ever support your choice.

Surprise! Some parents who seem hostile to the idea of childlessness come around to their kids' choices eventually. Many people have been surprised to find their parents or grandparents are allies in their decision—older people sometimes feel like they had too many kids too soon, and understand their kids' desire to make different choices. Give 'em some time.

Rick, the software developer who's now in his 40s, got a vasectomy when he was 28. At the time, his family was upset and thought he'd made a big mistake. But, over time, they became more open to the idea of him not having kids because it fits with his "counterculture freewheeling" lifestyle—he met his current partner while literally stark naked at Burning Man. As his parents came to accept him as the member of the family who will never settle in one place or have mainstream politics; they have become more open minded about his decision to not have kids. "There's been a little bit of the older relatives wagging their fingers at me and saying, 'One day, you'll want to settle down, too' but, so far, that hasn't happened," says Rick.

11. People don't *not* get pregnant accidentally.

While it's alarmingly easy to accidentally make a baby—half of all pregnancies in the United States are unintentional—staying baby-free is tricky.

There are many types of birth control, from condoms at the corner store to prescription birth control pills, but it's sadly normal to have trouble scrounging up enough money for birth control. Studies show that 99 percent of American women use birth control at some point, but that one in three have struggled to pay for it. Here's the good news: Federal funding under the Title X program covers the cost of birth control for low income women, which you can obtain at many clinics nationwide, including any Planned Parenthood. Plus, Barack Obama's Affordable Healthcare Act says that insurance companies have to cover the cost of birth control. For people who do not live near a clinic, or who make more than the "low-income" qualification but don't have insurance, birth control costs several hundred dollars a year. The cheapest, most effective forms of long-term birth control are intra-uterine devices (IUDs) and sterilization through a vasectomy, tubal ligation, or hysterectomy.

Slipping up has high stakes. Accidental pregnancies can create major fissures in relationships.

"I've seen it ruin marriages," says Ellen, the therapist. "I have a client that when she and her husband got married, one of the requirements was that they not have kids. She accidentally got pregnant and decided she really did want to keep the baby. He was so resentful and felt like he was manipulated."

12. **Pregnancy isn't just a lady problem.**

This should be obvious, but if you're a guy who's ardent about not having kids, you're responsible for making sure your partner doesn't get pregnant.

Statistics show that dudes don't play an equal role in using birth control, and the world would be a better place with fewer unwanted babies if they did. That means inquiring about whether your female partners are on birth control, insisting on using a condom if they're not, and considering getting a vasectomy if you're 100 percent sure you never want kids. That might seem drastic, but an increasing number of young guys are getting the snip. It's also worth noting that vasectomies don't have the hormonal side effects of most types of lady birth control.

"I feel great. It has taken a huge stress out of my and my partner's life," says PJ, a 28-year-old bike mechanic who got sterilized when he was 25. "The Pill was absolute torture for her. This was just like 'snip snip' and it's done."

Hiker Lint, meanwhile, has found sterility to be an excellent pick-up line.

"My vasectomy is one of the very first things I use," says Lint. "Okay, I meet a girl. Potential relationship. 'Hey, I have a vasectomy, you'll never get pregnant with me.' If she reacts negatively, phew, I don't have to worry about getting involved with someone who has completely opposite beliefs from me. Whereas if she's like, 'You have a vasectomy? Cool.' Then, well..."

13. There's some resistance to sterilizing people under thirty.

Though it's obviously the most reliable form of long-term birth control, young, childless people report that it can be tough to find someone willing to sterilize them. Lint and Hanna both decided to get sterilized in their mid-twenties.

When he lived in Ohio, Lint called several doctors to find one that would even see him for a consultation about his vasectomy because he was under 30.

"Every urologist I called, once they found out my age and that I haven't had kids, would just hang up on me," says Lint. After calling around, Lint eventually found a Planned Parenthood doctor who was happy to go through with the procedure.

Hanna, meanwhile, has not yet been able to find a doctor willing to sterilize women under 30. When she was twenty, Hanna's doctor told her that she didn't qualify for tubal ligation until she was 21... then, when she turned 21, the doctor bumped the age up to 25, and then 30. In the end, Hanna reluctantly used birth control pills and then got an IUD, which promises infertility from five to twelve years, depending on the type.

14. Some people do regret not having kids.

The biggest question young, baby-free people get is: "But won't you regret it?" And they're right! One out of five women who get their tubes tied when they're under 30 express some sadness over the decision. It looks like turning 30 really is some sort of tipping point, because a much lower number (six percent) of women over 30 who get their tubes tied express regret.

From talking with women's health doctors, the issue seems to be that people under 30 have more time for their lives to change drastically. They could go through a break-up or divorce or surprise themselves by finding a great partner that makes them realize they want children, or they can become economically stable enough to afford kids.

We can't talk about regret over not having kids without noting that there's a real double standard around baby regret. It's completely taboo to admit regretting having a child. I did a lot of digging, but can find hardly any surveys of parents about whether they regret having kids. The few studies that do exist come up with complicated results. A 1976 *Newsday* survey that showed about nine percent of Americans who have children say they regret the decision. A British study of 5,000 couples that Open University published in 2014 showed that childless couples reported they were generally happier than couples with kids, but that mothers were the happiest individuals of all. Meanwhile, a Princeton and Stony Brook University study of 1.8 million Americans found very little difference in the happiness levels of people with kids and people without kids, though parents reported experiencing bigger highs and lows.

It's not clear whether having kids or not having kids is really the key to a happiness, the numbers show it's more complex and personal than that. But for now, it seems like the only place you'll ever see people openly express regret about kids is online and in the therapy office.

15. People without kids have to seek out friends and community.

Every childless person I spoke with felt like the odd one out in some way or another because they don't ever want to have kids. It can be hard to make or keep friends as people around you start to have children. Kids tie their parents into communities—schools, summer camps, community plays—in a way that requires active work to make the same results happen if you're childless and seeking out places to get involved. Other people spoke about feeling left out of their office culture. "If I go out for drinks, I feel like I have to talk about my family," says

Tyler, a 31-year-old import specialist in Portland. "I do feel a real big self-consciousness. I do wonder, am I the only person who wants this?" Tyler mostly tries to avoid family conversations with co-workers and clients, but one thing that's helped, he says, is getting a dog. When people ask about children, he often winds up whipping out photos of his puppy, to ooo's and aww's. While they're not as obvious as, say, the Parent Teacher's Association, there are childless meet-up groups in most big cities. As with any subculture larger than two people, there are also a lot of childless communities online that swap advice and philosophies.

Last Thoughts

Talking to numerous people about their decision not to have kids inspired me to try and spend more time with little kids to see how I actually feel about hanging out with them. Luckily, my friends are full of babies. I signed up to help babysit a friend's two-year-old and made an active effort to hold friends' babies when they were proffered, instead of my typical response of cringing and shaking my head wildly. The verdict? My initial response to babies is still pretty much, "*Aaaaa!*" But seeing my friends manage well as parents makes me more able to imagine myself as a parent someday. Talking with all these people about their decision not to have kids made me feel less crazy and was a great affirmation that if I decide to not have children, there are strong communities of people who I can look to for friendship and support.

Right now, I completely agree with the logic and feelings of the childless-by-choice people I interviewed. But while I don't feel an urge to have kids, I don't feel committed to not having kids either. I'm going to stay open to the possibility of having a baby for at least the next few years—the important thing is to make sure I'm honest with my partners and let them know that if they're dead-set on a baby, I'm maybe not their girl. Who knows? Maybe I'll turn 35 and my long-silent uterus will leap into action.

WENDY-O MATIK

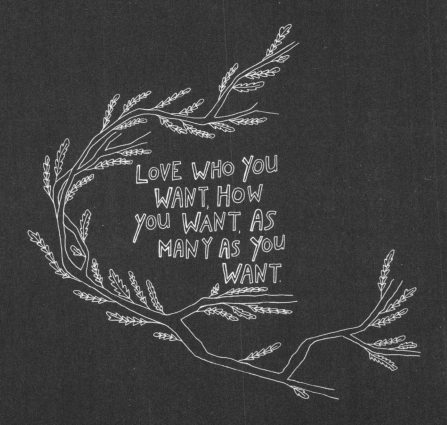

LOVE WHO YOU
WANT, HOW
YOU WANT, AS
MANY AS YOU
WANT.

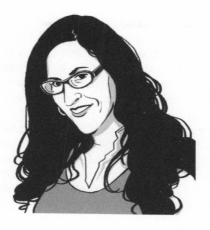

I waited a month for Wendy-O Matik's book to come off the library hold list and then gobbled up the slim volume, Redefining Our Relationships, *in one quick weekend. The personal, gushing guidebook to how the 40-something Bay Area "radical love warrior" approaches relationships struck my heart and stayed there. For many years, she was an archetypal punk, coming of age in Santa Cruz punk clubs, covered in tattoos, and denouncing marriage. While I'm used to punks being a little prickly and standoffish, during our conversation Matik was downright giddy. These days, Matik prefers work boots to combat boots and lives on Northern California ranch land, where she gets her hands dirty and punctuates nearly every sentence with a happy exclamation mark, even as she talks through the tricky feelings around feminism and choosing not to have children.*

Stick To Your Guns

I've always known I wouldn't have kids.

I had dreams when I was in high school that I was not ever supposed to give birth. I felt I had a mission in life and I didn't know what it would be, but I always knew it would mean I wouldn't be able to have kids. I would need to be, in some ways, selfish and not be able to sacrifice all that time and energy for children.

I grew up with the message that women's greatest role and their greatest purpose in life is to have kids. I always rebelled against that. I was in the punk scene, in a scene where we were always questioning authority and the media and I went right along with that. I was like, "Yeah, I don't need anyone to tell me that the only thing that's going to make me happy is a man, a white wedding, and having children." I knew that being somebody's wife wasn't going to make everything perfect.

It's not easy going against the grain, but that's all I've done all my life. I've dressed weird and taken the judgment for that. I'm bisexual, I've always been out about my queerness, and I've taken some heat for that. I've got a lot of tattoos. I've brought home girlfriends who look like men. My mother has been put through the ringer.

But at some point you tune out the criticism and the judgment. You tell yourself that you live true to your own values and ideals and you know it's going to be harder. It would be easier if I could just be monogamous and get married and have kids. It would be easier if I could just conform to be how everyone thinks I should be. But I can't live that way. I would be unhappy. I want to stay true to my values and this is the direction that I've headed.

You Can Be A Punk Without Dreadlocks And a Great Person Without Kids

I don't dress up anymore. I don't bleach my hair anymore, I took out all my piercings, I shaved off my dreadlocks. I had my dreadlocks for eleven years, they were past my butt; I had other people's dreadlocks sewn into my dreadlocks. I was just done. I said, "I'm a punk because of who I am and the way I think, not because I go to all the shows and wear all the clothes." Underneath, I'm the same person who is careful about what messages I listen to.

Even when I watch movies, they carry these messages: Your life has no meaning if you don't get married and have children. These messages make you hate yourself if you don't follow them. I try to always check in and remind myself, "This is my life, I get to do it the way I want to do it. I can even make mistakes."

Sure, I have relationships with children. A lot of my friends are single moms and I met their kids when they were two and three years old. I have beautiful relationships with them right now. I can come over to their house and say, "How's school? Do you have any boyfriends or girlfriends?" If they're in crisis, maybe they think to call me because they know I won't judge them. It's more like an aunt role.

I'm just not a baby type person. I'm an old people person. I have a lot of friends in their 70s and 80s. The way some people are with babies, that's the way I am with old people. I like hugging them and pinching their cheeks. I've always been that way.

You Have To Carve Out Freedom

Being a child was not a happy time for me—I grew up with a physically violent dad. I have some memories that are happy, but I remember being traumatized as a kid. I remember being scared a lot, crying a lot, being fearful of my dad. I have a unique relationship with my dad because in addition to him clearly having anger issues, he was also this profoundly loving teacher for me. I worshipped my dad, I was a daddy's girl. I walked in his shadow everywhere, even though I knew I risked being slapped, kicked, or spanked.

So I don't have this idea of childhood as so easy and fun and great. I grew up thinking, "This is awful and hard and painful and I didn't even ask to be here."

I think people sometimes have kids or get married for not the right reasons, like, "Oh, I'm supposed to do that." I don't want to live a life where I just do what I'm supposed to do. Of course, I pay my bills and I conform in certain ways, but that's just because I'm supposed to play by certain rules. But there are some rules I can break! And I'm going to push those.

Being in the punk scene, questioning war, and the government and all the influences that patriarchy has on women's reproductive rights, I was like, "You know, I do have a choice. And what I want to choose is freedom."

How I carve that freedom out is up to me. No one's going to hand me freedom on a platter, the freedom where you go against the grain and say, "I'm going to take the harder road. I'm going to choose polyamory and not having kids." I'm so fiercely independent. I've traveled the world with a backpack. I've hitchhiked and squatted in places. I've been a political activist. I've been arrested. I just don't see how I could have that lifestyle with a baby slung over me and having to breastfeed and getting no sleep.

I think I disappointed my family, for sure. No one said anything out right, but they hinted. Even now, my mom is like, "You would make such a good mother!" And I'm like, "No way. It's never going to happen."

It wasn't for me; I'm not cut out to be that kind of person. And maybe because part of me thinks I wouldn't be a good mother. I make a good dog owner.

Love Who You Want, How You Want, As Many As You Want

I just never liked one person. When I was in high school, I'd kiss someone and they'd say, "So you're my girlfriend now." I always felt weird. The message was: You meet someone, you like them, and then they become your boyfriend. I never liked that. It seemed confusing to me, alienating. I'd be at a party and I'd see two guys and I'd be like, "Oh, both those guys are cute" and I'd make friends with both of them and then maybe kiss one of them at one party and the other at another party. I didn't like to choose. But then that would cause problems. The one guy would find out about the other guy and he'd be like, "What the fuck is up with that?" And I'd be like, "What is it to you? My body belongs to me." But I never had the right language, I just made mistakes and people got hurt.

Whenever I tried to date someone, I'd say, "Can't we just be friends? If we do stuff, it's only because we're friends." I'd wake up in the morning and say, "See ya later" and we'd be friends again. I didn't want a boyfriend.

Even in college, I could tell guys wanted to get married, they wanted me to be their wife. It was the weirdest thing. I would be like, "I love you, I want to see you, I like sleeping with you, but I'm not going to have your baby or wear a white wedding gown, don't even go there. I'm 21, I don't even know what I'm going to do next week." In terms of my sexuality, I wanted to try everything. Hmm, sleep with someone who's into BDSM? Okay, I'll try that. I didn't like it? Okay, how about sleeping with two guys? Whoa, that was intense, I don't think I want to do that again. You know, I just wanted to try things and I didn't think having a steady boyfriend or girlfriend was a good idea.

In my twenties, there was no word "polyamory," there was just: You guys are freaks.

There was no internet, there were no support groups, there were no workshops. I started calling it "open relationships," but that's just something I made up when I was 23 or so. Even now, a lot of my monogamous friends don't know how to support me.

It's a subversive way of being in the world. We go against patriarchy, religion, everything our society has told us we're supposed to do. As women, we're supposed to be quiet and obedient and have babies and do what our husbands tell us to do. And I say, "Fuck that." I'm not talking about the theory or concept of feminism, I'm saying, I am a woman who's free to do anything she wants with her body—anything that is safe and doesn't hurt anybody—I am free to love who I want, how I want, as many I want.

Integrity, honesty, communication, and consent are at the core of any relationship. You might put on a business suit, you might do a corporate job to pay your bills, but when you go home and make love to whomever you want to make love to, you are embracing pure activism. You're not just sitting around letting people decide for you how you should be happy.

People are very judgmental. I think they're envious, like they see you having fun, enjoying yourself; you're not just stuck at home with the same person. You're doing whatever you want to do. You get in a van and go on tour, you meet someone new and spend a week with them, you have another boyfriend and people know about it. My best friends were all, "We don't understand it, we don't know how you do it, but we see you're happy and we support it."

You're Going To Make Mistakes, Together

I did get married once, but I'm not married now. It just wasn't part of my identity.

At 23, I met the guy I stayed with for thirteen years. I sat him down and said, "I'm crazy about you. I've had a crush on you for two years. I love your band. I love your music. I love you as a person. But, I have to tell you: I'm bi. I'm always going to desire other women. I don't know how to do relationships the way other people do. I need to be free. And if you call yourself an anarchist, if you call yourself a feminist, if you believe in the empowerment of women, then you need to uphold my right to be free. I'll uphold your right to be free. And it's going to be hard, because we're going to make mistakes and we're going to hurt each other. But I want you to know, if you give me total freedom, then I'll stay with you."

The thing we kept saying to each other was that we didn't have to break up just because we had a mistake. We can just say, "Wow, this is really painful, this is going to take a lot of time to process and renegotiate." It just took a lot of stumbling along.

You don't have a handbook that says: Do this and you'll have a fail-proof, sustainable relationship no matter what. No, every single relationship will be different, every single agreement will be different, and all along the way until you stop seeing that person, you will be renegotiating those agreements. Forever. Because what you desire in your twenties might be very different from what you desire in your 30s, in your 50s, and 80s. You need to redefine your relationship to fit your idea.

If you can wrap your mind around the idea that there's never one easy formula, it's trial and error, then you can sign up and have two people on board to create something sustainable and long term.

In our fifth year of being together, he started asking me to marry him. I said no for five years. He kept pushing it and talking about it and bringing it up. I was like, what's the point, who cares? I'm committed, I'm here. I live with you! But it was important to him. I felt like he was someone who shared the same values as me and if this was something that was going to make him happy, why couldn't I be more flexible? I started asking myself deep questions: If I love this man and this is what's going to make him happy, I think I can try this thing. It's something I cried about for a year. Even when I said yes, I found reasons to change my mind and cry. He kept being patient with me and eventually we had a wedding, a simple thing in the backyard. I wore a silver prom dress.

Marriage is an institution that's not afforded to everybody. It's a privilege to get married when my gay friends can't get married. It's a political act. I always held that ground. I'm a feminist, I believe in gay rights, and if gays can't get married, I can't get married.

Also, there's the whole ownership thing. I don't want to be owned by someone, that someone else can now charge and make decisions for me. If you're in a poly relationship, it means you're always kind of single, if you want to be. So the idea of putting a ring on my finger, what kind of message does that send to people? Oh, she's taken. But I got a ring.

It was the most painful relationship to lose, because he was my soulmate. He was the one person I would consider marrying and I did, for him. Now, we're still friends in spirit.

He met someone and wanted to be with her, but she wasn't into polyamory. She was into monogamy, and she gave him a choice: her or me. What kind of choice is that? You don't have a choice if someone isn't willing to share you. I was like, "Great! She can be with you these days of the week, I'll be with you these days of the week." I wrote her a love letter, I wanted her to be a part of my life, but she didn't want that. She felt threatened and freaked out by me. So I lost that relationship to another woman. But, you know, I knew about it. It wasn't like he lied behind my back or betrayed me.

When monogamous relationships break up, no one in their right mind says, "Oh my god, I knew monogamy didn't work." But when an open relationship breaks up, people say, "I knew it didn't work! Of course he's going to meet somebody and of course he's going to leave you." I don't see it that way. I see it as: People break up. People fall out of love, regardless of the relationship structure. At least in an open relationship, you don't have to cheat or lie about the people you get involved with intimately.

6.

On Never Getting Married

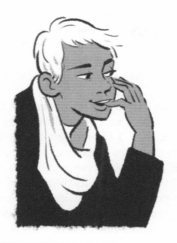

Marriage means success. It means you're happy. It means you're loved. It means you're on a stable track in life. It means you're not a total screw-up, at least.

Of course, that's all untrue. Truly happy marriages are more rare than we'd like to admit and there are plenty of married people who feel unsuccessful and off the rails. But that's the way we think of marriage. In America, no matter your background or politics, marriage is held up as an essential ideal. We all grow up singing the same little song about how life is supposed to go. "First comes love, then comes marriage, then comes a baby in a baby carriage."

Nigerian-born writer Chimamanda Ngozi Adichie stated that same idea in a slightly less-catchy way (until it became a sample on Beyonce's song "Flawless," anyway) in a speech: "Because I am female, I am expected to aspire to marriage. I am expected to make my life choices always keeping in mind that marriage is most important. Now, marriage can be a source of joy and love and mutual support. But why do we teach girls to aspire to marriage and we don't teach boys the same?" It feels like your relationship isn't "real" until it involves marriage—dating is aimless, unless marriage is the goal.

I've questioned a lot of aspects of my identity during my teens and twenties, but I've always assumed I'll get married at some point. First of all, I like a party. Secondly, that's just what's done. Everyone gets married at least once, right? Especially for women, your wedding is supposed to be the happiest day of your life—a crucial coming-of-age ritual that's necessary for starting the stable, adult, good-citizen phase of your life that involves a career and kids and making car payments.

It wasn't until I hit my mid-twenties in a long-term relationship with Carl that I started to have serious doubts about whether or not I should get married. I started to deeply fear how marriage could trap me. I had trouble with the concept of being with one person for decades, with cultural conceptions of what husbands and wives are like, and with other peoples' assumptions about what marriage means. I had this fear that by getting married, I would be forced into a more old-school, stereotypical mold of womanhood. I had this specific wifey nightmare: one day, I'd wake up in my mid-forties and be sullenly crying into a cake I was thanklessly frosting for his birthday. I would be bored. I would be dependent.

At the time, I was reading a lot of Raymond Carver, an author who pens somber stories where every relationship slowly grinds away people's lives, and Virginia Woolf, who speaks to the unique despair of frustrated ambitious women. Things looked bleak. The idea of deciding to become someone's wife, with all the historical and social baggage that word entails, began to appear terrifying.

As I've gotten older and become friends with married people and attended the weddings of some of my closest friends, I've come to understand that, like Adichie says, some marriages can be a source of joy and mutual support that help people become better humans over time—married people are not all resentful individuals who go around crying into cakes. I've rolled my eyes at some friends' wedding plans, sure, but other times when friends tell me they're engaged, I think, "Now that is a great idea." Personally, some days, I'd be crazy in love with my boyfriend and I'd think, "I could marry this person. It would be a thrill to wake up every day next to them, to laugh at their jokes every morning." Other days, I'd think the idea of me getting married is impossible.

But marriage has still never seemed like a genuine choice. People who don't get married in our society are treated suspiciously. I still feel like if I don't get married, I'll spend my whole life explaining the benefits of being an old maid. I'll be seen as too selfish to be in a "real" relationship. Some of the great appeal of a wedding is that it symbolizes for an entire community that someone who is not obligated to love you from birth has, indeed, decided to love you forever.

The question for me is whether marriage is an institution that can be bent and changed to be the way I want it. Or by getting married, would I inevitably be taking part in an institution that will change me to be more traditional? Is it really possible to subvert marriage?

The people I spoke with in this chapter have all asked that question and have come to one conclusion: no. Marriage will make their life less like the life they want to live. For all the positive aspects that marriage brings, it's not worth squeezing their relationships into the framework the institution offers. They're boycotting that husband-and-wife baggage, aiming to build their relationships on their own terms.

The Details

We're all familiar with the reasons in favor of getting married: endless, undying love, etcetera. But our romantic ideas about marriage are recent inventions. Until recently, marriage was a primarily economic arrangement between men. Romance was great, but marriage was intended to expand families' property and cement lines of inheritance. In the United States until the early 20th century, men legally gained ownership of any property owned by the women they married. Men also legally controlled the bodies of their wives—there was no such thing as rape within marriage, nor laws against domestic violence. Until the mid-twentieth century, it was rare for women to be able to earn enough money to support themselves into adulthood. As any Jane Austen fan could tell you, in previous generations, a woman without a husband (or a rich family) was in danger of financial destitution. In the 1950s, Simone de Beauvoir summed up this criticism, writing that marriage is prostitution in societies where women need to get married in order to keep a roof over their heads. Though women are still underpaid across-the-board today, marriage is no longer an economic necessity.

So while many modern marriages are wonderful, supportive, loving partnerships, marriage as an institution has some problematic roots.

More people are getting married later—or not at all—than ever in American history. For reasons I'm not entirely clear on but am already suspicious of, many studies of marriage keep track of marriage rates just for women. In 2011, 31 percent of adult American women were married, compared to 90 percent in 1950. That's a huge cultural shift. The average age of first marriage has ticked upward to 27 for women and 29 for men, from 20 and 23 in 1960. Americans these days are more likely to get divorced—about 40 percent of marriages end in divorce—and less likely than ever to get married at all.

Many commentators decry the increasing divorce rate, but I'm not too worried about it. The divorce rate reflects our changing ideas about what marriage means. Clearly, Americans are increasingly willing to recognize that marriage is not the right fit for every relationship—and are more able to call for a split when they want to.

Our cultural conceptions about what marriage means have changed dramatically over the past 100 years. And yet, marriage endures. Even with all the changes seen above, about 70 percent of American women have gotten married at least once. People seem to be more excited about throwing elaborate weddings than ever, with the average ceremony now costing just over $18,000. Millions of gay and lesbian Americans have fought for years for the ability to get married. Marriage is still an important symbol and a desirable civil right for the vast majority of Americans.

Those people who decide to reject the institution can teach us all a bit about how marriage has changed, where we should push it in the future, and whether marriage is the right choice for each of us.

One of the big reasons people decide to not get married is that they feel the institution can never be divorced from its patriarchal roots. Though many people these days write their own vows and nix the whole "obey thy husband" bit, the impact of two millennia of Judeo-Christian definitions of marriage seeps into the modern institution in ways that privilege the husband's identity and abilities over the wife's. For example, American women are expected to change their name when they get married and almost all of us do. Other traditional rituals, like being presented to your husband by your father, endure, too. Some people feel that no matter how you overhaul the wedding ceremony, you can never get away from the powerful and negative aspects of marriage's history.

Then there are people who have already been married and divorced and the experience soured them on the whole idea. My grandpa is in this camp. After he and my grandma divorced, he says he decided he never wanted to go through that kind of relationship again—now he's in his eighties and is content to be a world-traveling bachelor.

Whether or not you're dead-set on getting married, there is plenty to learn from people who have thought hard about the relationship change and decided it's not for them.

Ten Lesson to Learn from People Who Are Never Getting Married

1. **Not all good relationships lead to marriage.**

    This sounds obvious when I write it out, but it's the opposite of what we're taught, so it's a good place to start. Good relationships can end with breaking up. Good relationships can involve just kissing. Marriage is only the right choice for a specific set of circumstances. Ellen, a law office secretary, felt like marriage was the inevitable next step for her relationship with her boyfriend, since they'd been dating for a few years and bought a house together. They got married, but things changed and they wound up getting divorced—now she's convinced that their relationship would have been happier if they'd just kept dating and could have split up more easily, and she doesn't ever want to get married again.

2. **Marriage is a privilege.**

    Marriage is a civil right—but it's not afforded to everyone. One of the biggest reasons straight and bi people give for not getting married is that it's unfair to get hitched while many gay and lesbian Americans cannot benefit from marriage's legal privileges. "I would be really embarrassed to invite my queer friends to my wedding," says Patrick, who is bi and in a long-term relationship with a woman. "It would be rubbing it in their face."

3. **Marriage is clunky.**

Marriage is a heckuva lot of things: it's a tax system, it's a way to organize your family, it's a ritual with religious weight, it's a community recognition of your relationship, it's an expression of romantic love. Some people feel like they want part of the package—say, the tax benefits and community recognition—but not the whole institution. "The things I value in the idea of marriage are the things we have: commitment, recognizing our relationship, the explicit statement of working together, the assumption of a future together," says Megan, who has been with her partner for fifteen years and is unmarried. "All the important things are there, I don't feel like it's the government's business."

4. **Not getting married can be a nice way to define your own dynamic.**

When you get married, people will start to assume certain things about your relationship. Marriage entails a specific set of behaviors to many people and they'll assume you aim to abide by those, too. I remember my mom explaining how shocked she was after she got married to my father, John, that her in-laws started addressing letters to "Mr. and Mrs. John Mirk." Some of those assumptions you can work out through discussion—upon request, my grandparents started using her first name—but you'll still butt up against them again and again. People often want to pick and choose from marriage the parts they connect with and leave the rest behind. Not getting married makes it easier, in ways, to make your relationship look like whatever you want. Portlander Laura has been dating her boyfriend for over ten years—they have separate houses and sleep together a couple nights a week. She and her partner are content with their lives and their independent setups, but think that if they got married, there would be more pressure for them to have a more traditional arrangement and move in together. Laila, who is transgender, never wants to get married because they don't want to be simply replicating an institution developed by straight culture. Instead, Laila wants to craft a relationship from the ground-up that's free of sexism and traditional ideas about gender roles.

5. **Create your own rituals.**
One thing people miss out on by not getting married is a well-understood ritual for friends and family to recognize a serious relationship. Many people who decide not to get married make their own special events with their partners. For years, LGBT folks have held commitment ceremonies that look like weddings in everything but the legal paperwork. Many straight and bi people follow their lead. Instead of getting married, Megan and her boyfriend had a big ten-year anniversary party. Other people make a big deal out of holidays, like throwing a big Christmas or birthday party with their partner, to have some community recognition of their relationship. It can be rewarding to have some ritual, even if the whole wedding-bells thing isn't your style.

6. **There's no escaping the language of marriage.**
Everyone has to deal with the problem of the words "wife" and "husband." As musician Jonathan Richman croons to a slow beat in his song "When I Say Wife," "When I say 'wife,' it's cause I can't find another word for the way we be. But 'wife' sounds like you're mortgaged, 'wife' sounds like laundry." There's no universally guaranteed substitute, so if you're going to never get married, you'll have to come up with something. Many people use the words "partner" or "significant other" over "boyfriend" and "girlfriend," but—regardless of whether you're determined to remain unmarried or are just in a long-term relationship without getting married—figuring out how to express the gravity of your relationship to folks you've just met can be frustrating without the well-known verbiage.

7. **It can be nice to know your partner is not legally bound to you.**
Though many married people love how reassuring it is to have a life-long agreement to stay with their partner, the lack of legal ties creates a daily consent that many

unmarried people find important. The financial, social, and bureaucratic difficulty of getting divorced keeps some marriages together for longer than is healthy—splitting up when you're not married involves easier logistics. New York artist Kenan says his relationship with his long-term girlfriend feels more exciting and equitable because they're not married. "It's really good to feel like we are together because we want to be, not because we legally obligated to," says Kenan.

8. **Be skeptical of your reasons for wanting marriage.**
    There's no two ways about it, people will think you're kind of weird for not getting married. Marriage is a great and special step for many people. But because marriage is the default for our culture, there are a lot of forces pushing us to think it's the one and only route for life. If you do imagine a wedding in your future, think about what's motivating that desire. How much of a desire to get married comes from social pressure or the desire to make your life fit a specific plan? New Yorker Erin says she got married after she and her boyfriend were dating for several years because it just seemed like what was done. She was excited about the wedding at the time, but realized down the road that she was striving for an idea of how her life *should* look rather than what she actually wanted. Now divorced, she would rather have a long-term boyfriend than "slip" into marriage again.

9. **Marriage has a real religious legacy.**
    Whether or not you're religious, the way marriage functions in America is shaped by religion, for people who are strongly against organized religion. I attended a weekend-long wedding with a 60-something anarchist teacher named Baron, who was so opposed to organized religion that he not only never wanted to get married himself but refused to attend wedding ceremonies (he opted to play croquet rather than attend the ceremony that weekend).

10. **Get intentional.**
    Not getting married requires some serious commitment. We tend to reduce conversations about marriage to simple surprises, like "popping the question." Ideally,

marriage wouldn't mean popping anything, but having a mutual understanding of why you want to get married. Not getting married is the same way: you have to talk over with the people you're dating what you want to do and why. Falling into marriage out of habit and inevitability can be dangerous, but so can assuming that your partner will understand why you don't want to get married. Talk out what you want and why, including your issues with marriage and what you want your relationships to look like.

Last Thoughts

Marriage has a lot of baggage. I'm still not convinced that I want any part in the institution, but then I see good, smart friends of mine getting married and think maybe it can be alright, after all. I haven't come to any resolute conclusion about whether marriage fits into my politics, but right now, it doesn't have to. In theory, I think I'm opposed to getting married, personally. If I were to live completely in line with my abstract values, I would be vegan, run marathons, give away ten percent of my income to secular charities, always be punctual, and never get married. But, dammit, I'm always late, I love cheese, and there's no way I'm running 26 miles. Living as a practical citizen, I might someday get married despite the valid arguments against it, driven by sentimentality, love, and the tax code.

I admire the ways people have made their own enduring, successful relationships without marriage as well as how people have created happy, equitable relationships that involve marriage. I'm not sure whether I'll have the kind of relationship that leads to marriage. Four years into my relationship with Carl, one of my friends from college called to tell me she was getting married. I got the call at a bar, walked outside, and it was raining hard. She and her boyfriend, who are both farmers and musicians and all kinds of adorable, discussed getting married and she'd said, "That would make me the happiest girl in the world." I knew then, standing outside in the rain in the middle of winter, that if Carl asked me to marry him, I would not feel like the happiest girl in the world. I would feel nervous. I would probably say no. Not just because I was morally opposed to marriage's oppressive roots and discriminatory present, but because it would just feel wrong.

It's funny how being faced with a simple yes or no question can cut through the complexity to reveal how we actually feel.

BETTY DODSON

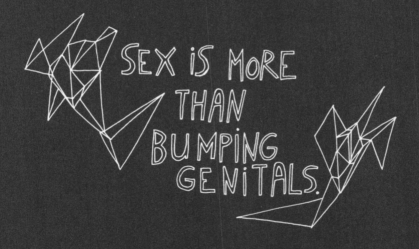

SEX iS MORE THAN BUMPING GENITALS.

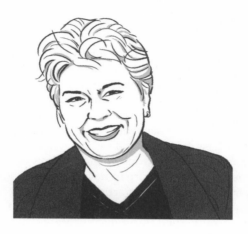

Betty Dodson opens the gray door of her Madison Avenue apartment and looks me up and down. "Hello, Amazon," she says, then offers to make me a drink. The 83-year-old sex activist is known for being direct, brassy, and unabashed in her language; during our 45-minute interview, she uses the word "fuck" seventeen times. The apartment where the legendary author of Sex for One *is host to masturbation workshops and is clean and sparse—Dodson's twenty-something live-in boyfriend Eric, moved out a few years ago. While still devoted to the physicality of life, in the past decade Dodson has discovered the thrill of the internet. Her main joy these days comes from answering teens' sex questions on her website, speaking without censorship or media filters for the first time in her life. Over vodka cocktails in her quiet home office, she talked about womanhood, religion, and the fake orgasms of the sexual revolution.*

Two Words: Honesty And Lube

Honesty is never natural. We all want to cop a plea or skirt the issue.

I came to New York to be an artist and tried the whole marriage thing and the monogamy thing and the sex was lousy. I didn't want to have a family and my husband agreed and then as soon as we got married, changed his mind. Everyone was having children and [long, angry sigh] it's hard to be different. Back then, I was much more traditional. To break these rules and deal with your family and friends— everyone's got a very strong opinion on how to live your life.

I never had the desire to have kids. Ever since I was a little girl, I wanted to be an artist. I did not want to be a wife and I did not want to be a mother. I helped my mother raise my little brothers and I saw what her life was like. Thankless. Oh my God. You want to talk about the most important job in the world? Raising a child. And we treat it like shit.

My husband finally came home one night, it was my birthday, we were having dinner at my favorite Japanese restaurant, and he said, "Oh I don't know how to tell you something." And I said, "What?! Spit it out!" And he said, "I fell in love with my secretary." And I said, "What? Just fuck her! Have an affair!" I thought that would be good because it would get him turned on. He was terrible in bed, a premature ejaculator. But every once in a while, he could fuck like a dream. It would be better to have it always bad or always good, but to have it be mostly bad and sometimes good, ugh. I would say to my therapist—I was in therapy— I'd say, "It's a breakthrough! We're having our breakthrough moment!" And then, nope, back to the preemie.

And of course, I was inhibited as much as he was. Oral sex? Nope. Manual sex? Nope. But sneaky masturbation, that got me through marriage.

I left a fabulous art career. I was good, I had two successful art shows. And the next thing my mother knows is I'm running masturbation workshops? My mom, she lives out in Wichita, she says, "Betty Ann, have you lost your mind? What do you mean they don't have orgasms? That's absolutely natural." It was natural for her; she was orgasmic.

There's a whole other aspect to that—my father was not circumcised. It's a whole different fuck when you're with an intact man. The foreskin is moist, it keeps the whole glans sort of satiny and soft, they can glide, not do the friction fuck. Don't forget to use lots of lube. Lube! Lube is the number one sex toy in America as far as I'm concerned. I would never have sex without anyone without additional lubrication.

You Can't Fix Your Hair During A Genuine Orgasm

I was part of the sexual revolution. I was going to sex parties and watching people have orgies and *whoa*. The women were all faking orgasm and the men were all cumming. It was clear to me. The women were all [Betty launches into a flamboyant physical reenactment of an orgy] "Uh! Uh!" then fixing their hair and the men were all [thrusting] "*uhh uhh!*" The women were all frilly and fluffy and concerned about how they looked. It was not acceptable. Absolutely not acceptable. It was so unfair! For the guys to be cumming and for the women not to be. They had no idea what an orgasm is or how to have one. And it starts with masturbation.

I got involved in the feminist movement and then I found out the feminists didn't want to deal with sex either. Still don't.

I want women to have independent orgasms. I want them to understand their bodies. I don't want them to go out into the world and let some well-meaning but stupid little jackass who doesn't know what they're doing fuck 'em. Teen pregnancy! They don't have any information. We send our little girls out into the marketplace totally unarmed, totally helpless. They don't have information, they don't have birth control, they're drenched in stupid ass religion!

Right now, we have a whole slew of teenagers coming up the pike who have been raised on abstinence only. And they are fucking. They are having sex. And it's penetration sex— they're either giving blowjobs or taking it up the ass. Making the man happy and not having anything for yourself? That's as ancient as the Bible.

It's gotten worse since the sexual revolution. We went into this religious mode. Look at Bush and company. We're still carrying on with the religious freaks.

I don't talk too much about it, but I honor the goddess of sexual love and abundance, and I'm an atheist. I respect the ancient religion, back when we had things worth worshipping: sex, life, and celebration, the stuff that was never written down. But if you go back and look at the art, she's there, she's everywhere. We are the power. We give birth. And boy does that piss mankind off. Damn!

Keep Fair & Keep Moving

In my seventies, with Eric, it was perfect. He wanted to be an apprentice and great! I was more than happy to teach him. I'm proud of him; he's doing well. It was the perfect time for me to have a live-in love affair. In your seventies, it's not like you want to go out every night and fuck everyone you can get your hands on. That was my forties. Fifties, menopause, meh. I took a break from penetration and hung out with the lesbians, the leather dykes. But I got bored with that, too, I don't want to always have a role and negotiate everything.

Revisiting heterosexuality was, in a way, novel. I hadn't done it for so long. Only this time, I had the power. In ways, it was like I was the husband and Eric was the wife. I got the whole picture of what that was like and it's very unbalanced. He who makes the gold makes the rules. Unless you're both working, earning an income, and putting it into a pot.

My challenge was not to abuse my power. So there were times when it got close to that, I would want him to do something differently. But I would always sit down and negotiate and I would always thank him for his work. Eric was working for me, so I was his boss, his teacher, his roommate, his lover. It was insane. I would never, ever recommend anybody do that. It was crazy! But I loved him and I loved it and we had a great ten-year-run. The last few years were rocky, I could tell he needed to move along.

It takes ten years to master any art form. He had all my information. If he kept hanging around, I would be crippling him. He would have been stilted. That's what should happen with relationships and marriages. A lifetime? Crazy! We change, we shift, we alter. Forever and forever until death do us part? That's like going to jail with a life sentence. Our relationship was fine for the time that we did it, but then he needed to move along. And he needed to be with an age-appropriate woman. You can't fuck granny for the rest of your life.

You Need Your Own Space

I would never say "sleep with" someone. I would never sleep with anybody. I'll have sex with someone, but I'm not going to sleep with someone. If they want to come over here and have sex, they have to leave. If they have to stay over because they're from out of town, they have to stay in the other room.

I had a bed to myself until I was 29. Boyfriends always wanted to sleep over, but they always wanted to fuck first thing in the morning and I wanted to wake up and brush my teeth and have my own space and my own time. As an artist, I always had something on the easel that I couldn't wait to get back to. And then, as a writer, I couldn't wait to get back to where I left off. So I didn't want someone hanging around. We'd have a date, he'd come over, we'd have sex, buh buh buh. My day is my own!

I always need to be alone. You need solitude; you need privacy.

I'm less likely to engage in partner sex these days, just because of my age. I'm not going to do it with an age appropriate man or woman. They're half dead! So it's going to be somebody younger, which means they'll have to be open minded.

I do occasionally have sex with people these days, I'm open to it. Last night, I got picked up in a restaurant by this rather attractive Chinese man. Tall, good looking guy, articulate. We had this marvelous conversation; we took down each other's phone number. He's 50 and he knows I'm 80. I think I'll wait and let him call me. I saw he had a wedding ring, not that that means anything.

I can have sex with someone out of curiosity. I don't need to be in love. Fifty-year-old Chinese man? Who's in the computer world? Hm. Smart!

Sex Is More Than Bumping Genitals

I'm branching out to where sex is much more than bumping your genitals together and [reenacts a gross makeout scene] *nom nom nom* slobbering and kissing *nom nom nom*. I've done that for thousands of years it seems. It has to be more of an intellect, it has to be more of a challenge, it has to have more of a meaning. Procreative sex? [Yawns]

Thinking about sex, drawing about sex, writing about sex, answering questions about sex, lecturing, talking; that's all sex! You think sex is just fucking with genitals! Oh please, darling, that's such a small part of it.

Women don't understand their bodies. They don't look at their pussies. They don't know what their cunts are made of. They don't know where their clitoris is. They think they have to cum from vaginal intercourse. I've been talking about this same stuff my whole life and I never get bored. Not when I get an email like—I had this woman show up on Saturday who said she had her first orgasm at 25 after reading my instructions on what to do. Are you kidding me? Do you know what kind a reward that is? 25 years old and never had an orgasm in this world where we're surrounded by sex sex sex!

On the website, *oooo, we're cookin'*. We're putting out the information that these kids really need. I get up in the morning and I can't wait to get to the computer. I'm 83 years old and I am dealing with thousands of people. I've been censored all my lifetime and now I'm not. My bliss and my ecstasy are helping these kids find some answers to their sex problems. Everything about that is orgasmic to me.

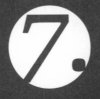

Knowing
When To
Split

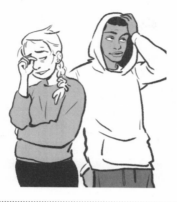

The hardest part of being in a relationship is knowing when it needs to change.

When Carl and I went to counseling, finally, one winter, the counselor asked me what my biggest fear in the relationship was. I knew immediately: that I'd feel trapped in a relationship that was making me go crazy.

It's not always noble to stay in a relationship—certainly not if it's making your future look darker, not brighter. I want a relationship that gets better over time, not worse. But breaking up feels like failure. The primary way we judge the healthiness of relationships in America is by their longevity. We clearly need some better definitions of success.

We'd been good at talking over our feelings and pushing each other to be more honest, but it took years for me to understand that Carl and I should not be dating. After all the discussion, the sad answer struck me like a thunderbolt.

I wrote in my journal, "I never want to have sex with Carl again." I wrote the words in ink, but I didn't want them to be true. They were terrifying. It knew it wasn't a changing feeling, an attraction that would come and go. It was a deep-down in-my-gut knowledge. I was unhappy. So was Carl.

I was furious with myself; the realization felt unfair and irrational. And I was right—it is unfair when relationships between great people don't work out. Carl and I line up on all the big important stuff that matters, like our curiosity about the world and our love and respect for each other. If our relationship were a math problem, it would pencil out perfectly. But attraction isn't rational and neither is mental health. There's some magic to those realms, some unsolved primal science that doesn't play by the rules we want it to.

I knew from all my conversations with people in different types of relationships that I needed to have a baseline of sexual attraction to my partner. Never wanting to have sex again—that was a deal breaker. The fact that we'd both been unhappy for a long time, despite intentionally working to be happier and healthier—that was a deal breaker, too.

It took a long time for me to feel like it was okay if we broke up—that it wouldn't mean *I'm* broken. I wanted to be a success story: the smart people who could build communication that was good enough to talk their way through any problem. Our love would be enough to get us through thick and thin. We'd still be joking with each other on our deathbeds.

I kept the knowledge inside for a long time, as a secret I wasn't planning to tell. I wouldn't say I wanted to break up, but I schemed to tell Carl a softer version of the truth. We'd ease into the process with some white lies. I went around lining up the break-up logistics. I found a sofa to sleep on. I saved money to pay a deposit on a new place to live. I looked through real estate listings and found a nice place. Then I told Carl that I thought I should move out but that we shouldn't break up.

But he pushed me, like he always does, telling me that he could feel I was holding back. He could tell I was silently planning something big.

"You not trusting me is more hurtful than anything you could say," he told me.

So I blurted it out, all the things I'd been afraid to say. I told him I never wanted to have sex with him again and that we were both unhappy and that I thought we should break up.

He absorbed it all and thanked me for being honest. Then we went for a walk and got milkshakes. We stayed together for a few more weeks as I moved out.

The night we broke up, I laid on the cold kitchen floor in my new house. All I could conceive of doing was listening to music and staring at the ceiling. Eventually, my roommate came home and turned on the lights. I told her what had happened and everything I'd done wrong.

"Well," she said. "The good news is I bought a waffle maker. We can make sadness waffles."

Soon, the kitchen was full of light and friends. We could laugh about things that had only recently been unnamable.

No matter what happens in my relationships, the things that hold true are honesty, friendship, and waffles.

The Details

Splitting up always feels messy and tricky and difficult and complicated. But, in the end, it comes down to one simple question: Do you want to stay in the relationship or not?

Figuring out the answer to that simple question is what takes lots of questioning, discussion, and work.

No matter how good you are at talking things out, not every breakup is going to go well. There are too many factors in play to guarantee that no one in the relationship will get mean or feel wronged. And no matter how well it goes, it's going to hurt. A lot of the tough work of breakups is logistical work. Agreeing on the concrete details of what to do about the house, the kids, and the possessions is the kind of hard decisions that make good feelings go sour. The specific logistics of finances, ownership, and custody issues, you'll have to figure out given your own situation. The goal of this chapter is to equip you to use your best judgment in these tough decisions. This chapter shares ways that people have determined the answer to the question of "should I stay or should I go" and how they've worked to create healthy lives for themselves and positive relationships with their former partners in the wake of breakups.

Along with that goal, the big idea I'm trying to wrap my head around is that breaking up is not failure. Whenever I break up, it means I'm diverging from a plan I liked at some point and it always involves saying goodbye to a lot of good things along with the bad. But in almost every relationship in my life, at some point, breaking up will be the smartest and bravest choice. Breaking up means the people in the relationship aren't going along with the status quo—unless it's an impulsive and poorly considered mistake, it means that you are thinking about what you want and need and speaking up about it. That's a good thing, at its heart, though it's hard to see it that way amid all the chaos of heartbreak.

We have a simple image for what breaking up looks like: ice cream, sofa, uttering spiteful words about your ex. But it's not like a pint of ice cream can cure all wounds. Just like relationships, breakups look all sorts of ways. They can mean you don't have sex anymore or that you stop speaking to each other. Or splitting can up can mean that you become non-sexy best friends instead of romantic partners, or acquaintances who are always happy to see each other around. Your lives can diverge completely or you can evolve into a new kind of partnership. Ideally, they're a positive change that both people eventually agree is the right idea.

20 Lesson From People Who Have Split
1. You deserve to be happy.

Why does this sound so radical? Happiness is basic. It can be hard to recognize what in your relationship is grating on you and, if you've felt unhappy for a long time, it can feel impossible to decipher what parts of that unhappiness are due to your relationship and which are coming from within. This is especially hard if there's nothing concretely "wrong" with your relationship.

"I always looked down on people who were divorced," says erotica writer I.G. Frederick, who was married for nineteen years to a financially successful Republican fellow. "People who found out that we were getting divorced didn't get it; they thought I was crazy. They said, 'He doesn't beat you. He makes good money. What's the problem?'"

But the first step toward figuring out whether you should break up is figuring out what the points of conflict are in your relationship and considering the ways those are making you unhappy in the long-term.

Jan and her husband were best friends before they got married. Their wedding was a bow on the perfect life that she wanted to build for herself; a way of showing others that she was happy. But after about a year of marriage, she realized that she was walking through each day upset and on edge. At first she didn't even consider divorce—she and her husband had promised all their friends and family that their relationship was for life. "We stood up in front of 100 people and said we wouldn't do this," says Jan. "But I didn't want to spend my life cranky."

2. **Recognize what you need.**

In thinking about what's making you unhappy, it's helpful to figure out what you need from your primary partner. Think of needs like a value set. What are the values you want in your relationship? Portlander Ellen, who was married for six years before getting divorced, made a literal list of her needs. She would think about which of her needs were getting met and which were not, then write all that out, think it over, and discuss it in a "friendlier format" with her husband. For example, she needed a partner who could be deeply and openly emotional with her—that wasn't getting met, because she felt like her husband was rather icy when the conversation turned to emotions. "We couldn't get to the level of talking about ideas. I need a lot of intellectual stimulation. Can I get that from friends? I think I need it from my partner," says Ellen. I tried this, too, when I was trying to figure out what just didn't feel right in my relationship with Carl [See my handwritten list of needs on the last two pages of this book]. On the top of my list of needs is a partner who is curious and engaged in the world—that need was certainly met. I also need a partner who pushes me to be more honest and open up about my feelings—Carl did a great job of that. But also on my list of needs was having a partner with whom I enjoy having sex. That wasn't being met. Writing out what needs were met and unmet helped me develop a language to start talking about what was wrong, instead of just shrugging and saying, "I dunno, it's just not right."

3. **Think about who you are on your own.**

One big problem most people run into with relationships is a melding of identity between partners. After a long time building your life around someone, even thinking about not being in the relationship can feel like slicing off part of who you are. But in order to recognize what you need, you have to pull your head out of the sand a bit and look around at what's important to you as *you*, not as part of a unit. A big change in Jan's marriage came when her dad died. Mourning her dad became her number one priority and her relationship came second. "After being so 100 percent 'girlfriend' for a long time, it became a time where I was like my own person," says Jan. Taking time to consider her own priorities made her re-think the acceptable dynamics of her relationship.

4. **Articulate some deal breakers.**

This is another way of thinking about what your needs are and whether they're being met. Are there things in your relationship that are absolutely not working? Are they things that can change? How much time are you willing to be all-in on working to improve those things? If they're necessary for you to have, that's a deal breaker. For example, many people find sexual issues to be a deal breaker—if your libido has changed or you never really liked having sex with your partner to begin with, having a relationship that includes good sex could be a baseline that your relationship isn't meeting. For other people, communication styles can be a deal breaker. If every discussion is turning into an argument that leaves you all feeling frustrated, getting to a point where you can't talk through issues respectfully could be a deal breaker. For Jan, the real deal breaker was mental health. Her husband was bipolar and increasingly volatile. Jan came to understand that she didn't want to put up with his highs and lows for the rest of her life, to be tiptoeing around him in worry during the good times and trying to forget the hurtful things he said during the low times. "I didn't want an unstable life," she says. Having a mentally stable partner was a deal breaker for her (and many people).

5. **It's okay to change your mind.**

Okay. This is the tough part—to know that at some point you were excited about the relationship you'd mapped out (right? Maybe it was a long time ago) and to accept that your life isn't going to go as planned. Recognizing that plans diverging can feel like failure. After fifteen years of marriage, I.G. looked around at her life and came to understand that it wasn't what she wanted—after years of working toward getting the right house in the right neighborhood and building a good-looking marriage with her husband, it started to chafe. "We worked our whole lives to get to this point and then I felt trapped," she says.

6. **Build yourself a support system.**

Becoming a happy couple can be isolating. Everyone has

been guilty of this at some point: spending so much time with a partner that you leave your friends behind. This is the point where you pick up the phone and invest in friendships. Friends and family can help you sort through what you're feeling and what you need. Know who's on your speed-dial for when you're feeling overwhelmed and need someone to eat misery ice cream with. If there are communities and parts of yourself that have fallen away as you've spent more time on your primary relationship (or, uh, watching Netflix on the sofa in said relationship) look around and see if you want to get more involved in groups and activities outside your little pod.

7. **Tell your friends the dark stuff.**
   Part of the isolation of being in a relationship is that you want your friends and family to like your partners, so there's a tendency to gloss over the bad stuff. There's a lot of pressure to present the image of a content couple and not discuss the things that rub you the wrong way about each other. But that can lead to you feeling like no one actually understands what you're going through. And they likely won't ever understand if you don't tell them. Find close friends or family members who you feel comfortable opening up to and pour it on out—push yourself to get vulnerable, you need people you can be honest with, not people you need to be polite around.

8. **Talking about feelings is damn difficult.**
   This is, for many people, the most terrifying act of all. If you really don't care about the person you're dating, you can skip this and just cut and run. A lot of people do this in the beginning of relationships—instead of telling a person why they don't want to keep dating, they'll just go "radio silent." But if you know your partner enough to be honest, once you've done some deep thinking and talking with friends about what you need, you've got to pluck up the courage to tell the person you're dating what you're feeling. This is the scary conversation, the one people dread, where you say the things aloud that you've been thinking through. From there, you can figure out how the relationship will change and evolve.

9. **You may try to commit some sabotage.**
   Instead of talking through her hostile feelings with her husband, Ellen went on Craigslist and sought out

an affair while he was out of town. "I was like, 'Holy shit, what did I just do?'" Then she hooked up with a coworker. The affairs were a red flag; she was hoping to create a concrete problem that she could point to as a reason why they should get divorced, rather than trying to articulate her complicated feelings of disconnect and anger. Her acting out didn't work. She told her husband about her affairs and said she thought they should call it quits—he forgave her and said he was up for working on the relationship. "The last thing I wanted to do was hurt him, but I was already not the person he wanted."

10. Try seeing a counselor.

Many people find it helpful to have a time and space to discuss issues in their relationship. For some people, a counselor provides time and space that's set aside to talk things through and it can lift a gloomy cloud off the rest of your time together. Other people come up with their own unique ways to create space for talking, like setting aside a morning where they always talk about issues from the previous week that they didn't want to bring up in the moment.

11. Make a plan.

It can be hard to visualize how a relationship could possibly end, especially if you live together and share income. So part of building your support system needs to be laying the logistical groundwork for what you'll do if you decide to leave. If you had to find a new place to live, where would you go? Should you start looking for a new place to live? Do you have the money to pay rent at a new place? If not, how can you get it? Are there things your partner provides—like a ride to work—that you'll need to sort out? These obstacles become the reasons a lot of people stay in relationships longer than they want to. In addition to the emotional complications, there are basic survival needs. This isn't about having one foot out the door, this is about making sure you're as safe, healthy, and stable as possible if you do decide to leave. But many people have dealt with all these obstacles. Finding good solutions for the most likely what-ifs will make breaking up look like a viable option and making a plan for yourself will make the whole process less stressful, if that's what it comes to. If you've got enough money in your bank account to pay for food and rent when you tell your partner it's over, you're a lot better off than some people facing a break-up. It takes a lot of courage to cut and run from a relationship, especially if you don't have a stable income.

12. Say the stuff you're afraid to say.

This only applies if you're feeling physically safe enough to be honest. But if you're both of stable enough temperament, many people find it helpful to lay all their cards on the table. Otherwise, many people end the relationship with a lot to say and harbor guilt and bad feelings or send inopportune text messages. Getting the feelings out is both a way to work through your issues honestly and a future-late-night-angry-text prevention plan. Ellen spent a long time in her marriage biting her tongue. When they were considering divorce, she learned how to speak up about how she felt and it's helped the couple maintain a good relationship as friends. "Now I err on the side of saying too much. I listen more and figure out how to convey my message in a way that doesn't shut him down," she says.

13. When you want to get out, get out.

There's only one way to say it: when you gotta go, you gotta go. If you've evaluated your needs, talked through them with your partner, built yourself a support network, and feel like the right decision is ending the relationship, it's the right decision. "The only thing I would have done differently is leave sooner," says IG, who is now in her fifties. "I wouldn't have told my 29 year old self to get out, I would have told my 40 year old self to get out. I don't regret having married him, I don't regret having left him either."

14. Someone has to make the call.

At some point, someone needs to actually say they want out of the relationship—and stand by that decision. Computer programmer Rick remembers sitting in the living room with his wife, talking about how they were miserable and fighting all the time. One of them said that they could get divorced. "I actually felt better. I realized, 'Oh, we're not doomed. Worse case scenario, we could get divorced,'" says Rick. When Portlander Ellen was debating whether to stay in her six-year marriage, she took a weekend and went to San Francisco by herself. She had a lot of fun hanging out in the city with friends.

When she got back, Ellen and her husband went straight from the airport to marriage counseling. "The counselor asked if I was willing to work on the marriage," she recalls. "It was one of those one-word answers: 'No.'"

15. Activate that support system.

This is when your friends make you waffles and you sleep on their sofa bed because you're too sad to go home. Recognize that you'll be feeling alone and isolated and reach out to people. In addition to leaning on friends for emotional help, activate your own internal support system—this is a crucial time to keep yourself busy and healthy. Get enough sleep. Get some exercise, even if you haven't in forever.

16. You will grieve.

Everyone mourns a relationship in their own way. Jan spent a month on the sofa, forcing herself to go to work everyday but spending a lot of time thinking through things by herself, with her pets and a couple close friends for company. Other people like to go out and whoop it up, reveling in flirting with new people. Recognize that you'll be grieving for a while; whatever your style is, know that you're in an emotionally vulnerable place where you might make bad, impulsive decisions (the dreaded break-up haircut, for example, or sleeping with someone you don't even like). Lean into that support system.

17. It's okay to be angry and sad.

Sometimes, breaking up feels like barfing. You may also feel so much better afterwards that there's a tendency to say, "I'm totally great!" But many people report a false sense of being okay—you don't have to pick yourself right up and be perky. Find positive ways to deal with your anger and sadness after a breakup, so drudging through those feelings doesn't become consuming. Many people deal with that sadness by making art or writing, or pouring their restless energy into exercise. Allowing yourself time and space to be upset is a skill.

18. You don't have to be friends.

"I wish I hadn't tried to be so cool about everything. I wish I had decided sooner that we didn't have to be friends." says Jan. She and her ex-husband had a lot of mutual friends. Since they'd been the perfect couple in some peoples' eyes, she wanted to be the perfect broken-up couple, too: the people who can hug each other and hang out at parties together, no problem. Instead, she found that seeing him was emotionally draining and knowing he would be somewhere kept her away. Just like in a relationship, during a breakup, recognize what you need and think about how to fill that need. Do you need the person to apologize for some specific actions? Consider telling your ex that's what you need to make your hurt and anger lessen. Do you need time alone to think through your feelings? You can definitely make that. Do you need to feel sexy again? Dancing cures all. Each situation is different, so give yourself permission to say you don't want to see someone for a while or to communicate that you're not up for being friends. In situations were one or both of you is hurting deeply, it helps to have clearly articulated guidelines about when and whether you're allowed to contact each other. If you're both up for talking, great! Go get dinner. But if not, make it known rather than simmering in resentment whenever they call or you cross a boundary yourself.

19. **But you don't have to be enemies.**
   One big problem with the way relationships are portrayed in pop culture is that exes always have an axe to grind. Whether they're jealous, lecherous, or out for revenge, they're certainly not to be trusted. In real life, people have all sorts of relationships with their exes. You've been through a lot with each other and likely know each other pretty well—that kind of connection with someone is worth holding on to and valuing, if the hurts between you aren't too deep. While Jan and her ex-husband are no longer speaking, Ellen and her ex-husband have a solid friendly relationship where they work together on house projects and keep up to date on each other's lives. IG and her husband are pretty indifferent toward each other, since their lives have gone in different direction, but she says there's a warmness between them rather than a hostility. If it feels right to you, don't be embarrassed about keeping the channels of communication open between you. Your relationship isn't necessarily ending—it's changing. If you can, respect your ex for who they are. It is helpful to tell your friends what kind of relationship you have with your ex—people will want to know whether it's alright to invite you both to the same events or whether they should try to only see

you separately. Getting practical with mutual friends about what you want from them helps makes the transition from dating to just-friends go more smoothly.

20. Moving forward, learn to trust yourself.

Dating is awkward and hard for anyone, but especially when you're trying to restart after being in an intensely focused relationship. If the relationship didn't go as planned, it can be especially hard to feel like you can have faith in future relationships or can trust yourself to know what you want. As corny as it sounds, breakups are often the way we learn what we want from our relationships, what we need from our partners, and our good and bad patterns in relationships. Take the time to recognize what created conflict, what needs went unmet, and trust in what you've learned. Plus, dating new people can be exciting, eventually. Says writer I.G., "The best part of being divorced is being in a relationship where I'm truly happy."

BREAK UP ACTION PLAN

You've just had the conversation. It's final. It's real. Here's what to in the next 24 hours.

1. Get out of the house. Pack your tissues and headphones and go for a walk around the neighborhood, catch the bus to a park, or go on a mini-roadtrip to your favorite coffee shop in the next town over. Staying in bed alone with the lights off listening to *Rumors* on repeat will just lead to wallowing, trust me. Fresh air is preferable.

2. Phone a friend. Schedule low-key things to do with friends for the next couple of days. Dinner plans with your closest friends will give you concrete things to look forward to and having some company while you watch a movie will feel like the nicest thing in the world.

3. Lose yourself in a story. This is your excuse to go buy that book you've been wanting to read, to see that cheesy movie you secretly want to see, or to watch your favorite *Star Trek* episodes again. There's a limit to this, of course, but turning your brain off for a bit while you devour some media can be a welcome relief.

4. Stay healthy. You might not feel like eating or sleeping, but you need those things. Go to the grocery store and buy your favorite healthy foods (plus chocolate) so that you'll want to eat them. Stock up on vitamin C, ginger, lemon, and other good stuff that keeps you strong, while you're at it. Go to bed at a reasonable hour and promise yourself you'll actually go to sleep instead of looking at the internet.

5. Exercise is magic. Exercise is the cheapest and most effective way to make yourself feel good. Go for a long walk, get running, bike to a friend's house, do some yoga. Your body will help you feel better.

Last Thoughts

Breaking up sucks. Every part of it is hard and sad. It can be necessary to wallow in that horribleness a bit. But what's not necessary is taking on the stigma of breakup and divorce. Because a relationship ends doesn't mean the relationship failed or that you failed as a person. Sure, there are people who break up for silly reasons (cup size, for example) and many people carry a lot of guilt about the way they treated a partner. But in the best-case scenario, breaking up means that the people in the relationship were up for thinking critically about their needs, their life, and their partnership and taking action to make their lives healthier and happier. That's the big picture—and in a world where no partner is perfect, it's a good one to embrace. Knowing how to quit a relationship and keep yourself healthy is a real skill.

For all that positive talk, I had a lot of days after Carl and I broke up where I moped around town, feeling like we'd failed. There were lots of ways that we wish we'd been better to each other. But, we've kept being honest with each other. We know each other better than almost anyone in the world. We're willing to work through the sad stuff to keep each other around. Over time, we've built a whole new relationship as good friends. Every day, we still get to give each other love and trouble.

TOMAS MONIZ

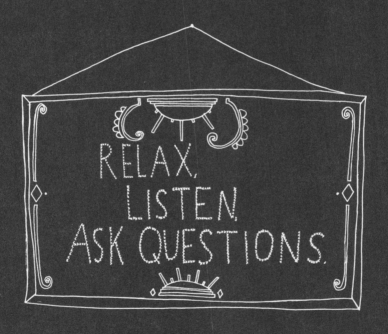

RELAX,
LISTEN,
ASK QUESTIONS.

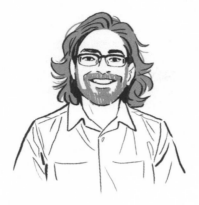

Rad Dad *magazine is a ray of light. While most of the parenting magazines that crowd the grocery store rack are about trends and new things to buy,* Rad Dad *asks big questions about politics and feeling good about what you do. The magazine was started by Tomas Moniz, a humble dude who lives in Berkeley and will happily tell you how much his kids make fun of him by sarcastically calling him "Rad Dad." Moniz and his wife Donna had their first child very young and spent the past decade navigating the tricky waters of raising open-minded kids while managing their own lives. Now a professor and father of three, Moniz is still in the constant process of figuring things out. We sat down for a slice of pie one spring day and talked about writing, family, and splitting up.*

Relax, Listen, Ask Questions

If it's the only parenting advice I give, it would be: Relax, listen, ask questions. It's the daily act of parenting.

I started *Rad Dad* seven years ago. I needed help. I didn't want to parent the way I was parented, which was a lot about shame, guilt, and control.

I wanted to find other people who were interested in being genuine. When I found my son watching pornography, you know, I don't want to shame porn. I want to have an honest conversation. I want to say, "I have looked at pornography, but I'm an adult." It was the same thing with drugs. To tell my son something like, "Don't do drugs, they're bad"—that's not genuine.

I need to ask myself, "What am I actually upset about? Why do I feel angry?"

There are moments that are crisis. Like my daughter had a party at my house when I was on tour with the *Rad Dad* book. She completely cleaned up, I wouldn't have known if the neighbor hadn't ratted her out. I had to think about why I was angry, and it was a couple things: One, that her boyfriend spent the night at the house and, two, that she lied to her mom and me. I asked her, "Do you think it was appropriate to do? Why didn't you just ask me? What were you afraid I would have said?" She was afraid I would have said no, and I told her, "Yeah, but that's my choice to say yes or no." These are moments that are few and far between. Mostly, it's trying to remember every day, during dinner, doing homework, to stay present in my relationship with her.

Parenting by denial is not a good thing. When we talk about sex, I'm like, "Don't have sex, here's condoms."

Give Your Kids The Skills To Ask Questions

With TV and YouTube, there's no way to monitor what they're watching. It's already a lost cause as soon as you start thinking about it. All I can do is give them the skills to ask questions.

Donna and I have been conscientious about bringing up sexism every time we have a chance to talk about it. Same thing with racism and homophobia. They get sick of talking about it but, hey, that's my job.

I had some great ideas, like no dresses in my house, no pink. But at some point, I let what happens happen.

I don't try to censor much. I try to model my own behavior. We didn't watch any movies with sexual violence in front of them, but whenever that stuff happened, it was an opportunity to have a conversation. When people make sexist comments in front of them, I mention it. I realized it was less about not letting them see things than when they do see things, having the skills to talk about it.

My mantra has been: If you're old enough to do it, you're old enough to talk about it. If you're old enough to watch a scary movie, you're old enough to talk about the violence. If you're old enough to wear makeup, you're old enough to talk about why you want to wear makeup.

A few months ago, we were talking about makeup and my daughter said, "When I don't wear makeup, I feel naked." And I said, "Whoa, that's really intense. Really? If you don't wear your eyelash stuff, you feel naked?" And she was like, "Yeah." And I didn't say anything else. I think they are shocked when they say that stuff, so they don't need me to reinforce it. They see it.

Let Your Relationship Evolve

Donna and I were together for fifteen years. We were babies together; we had kids when we were very young. She totally trusted me to parent.

We had an open relationship. When we were living together, Donna and I would just take turns dating other people, like you've got this Friday night, I've got next Friday. When we first opened up, we had all these rules to micromanage, but they fell away when we trusted each other. It was fun. I knew Donna was there for me, we were a priority, so that made it very easy.

It's harder being non-monogamous with people now, when you don't have that support. When I had a partner, there was a lot of trust and support. Now, when I have someone who I've been dating for a little while—you just don't have that shared, built-in history.

One of the mistakes we made is that we should have been more open with our youngest daughter about dating. Donna and I kept going as friends, really intimately, without mentioning to our kids that we were seeing other people. We worked so hard to have a good relationship that I think the reality of us not living together didn't fully sink in. In retrospect, I thought I had brought it up. But I never showed my dating to them, partly because my of respect for Donna, I kept that spot for her. So, the first time that my daughter met someone I'd been dating, she was a stereotypical terrible teenage child. It's almost laughable how horrendously mean she was to the woman I was dating.

When she moved out, I learned more about what I wanted. I repainted every room. We believe relationships can evolve, our relationship can evolve. We biked down the coast of Oregon as friends. That was the seal of our friendship. Now we basically share meals, one every couple weeks. We were very clear that we wanted to be co-parents.

We were joking that we're going to have a divorce party. You want to celebrate your relationship, you know?

It's rare to find a nonfiction work that approaches relationships from a sex-positive and open-minded standpoint. That's why, when I *have* come across books that promote healthy and critical ideas about relationships, reading them feels like an earthquake. Here is a reading list of books that shook me and shaped this book.

bell hooks' *Communion* is the place to start, because she notes the right place for all good relationships to begin: with loving yourself. I wish *Communion* were required high school reading, though I probably would have brushed it off as overly cynical when I was a teen. But if I'd taken the time to let the book sink in, I would have taken to heart hooks' insights that at the core of a lot of problems with our romantic relationships are our insecurities about our own value—and how our society is designed to make women, especially, question our worth.

Moving on from love to science, *Sex at Dawn: The Prehistoric Origins of Modern Sexuality* by Christopher Ryan and Cacilda Jetha dismantles the conception that there is one, true "normal" approach to sex and relationships. Their book brings together biological and anthropological research that upsets the idea that humans are naturally made for monogamy, instead showing how cultures throughout history have created their own unique ideas of what is a normal relationship. In a similarly academic vein, Erik Berkowitz's *Sex and Punishment: Four Thousand Years of Judging Desire* lays out how institutions—like religions and politically powerful groups—carefully construct cultural understanding of the acceptable ways to date, form unions, and have sex.

While *Sex at Dawn* and *Sex and Punishment* deal with interpersonal relationships on a centuries-long timescale, there are a few great books that document modern-day relationships that look different than the narrow spectrum of role models we see on TV. *The Ethical Slut: A Guide to Infinite Sexual Possibilities* by Dossie Easton and Janet Hardy is the classic that many people, including myself, have turned to for validation that our thoughts about dating are not as absurd as they seem. Wendy-O Matik's *Redefining Our Relationships* is a great first-person companion read to that book, a manifesto that reveals the problems and daily goodness Wendy-O found in her own feminist and non-monogamous dating life. Tristan Taormino's *Opening Up: A Guide to Creating and Sustaining Open Relationships* casts a broader net, looking at the logistical ins-and-out of open relationships in dozens of peoples' lives. *Opening Up* was certainly a model for this book and is a practical guide packed with useful questions for anyone thinking about what they want in their relationships.

The details of relationships are typically kept out of sight behind bedroom doors, so I appreciate the work that illuminates all the different types of relationships people make with each other. I like Arianne Cohen's *The Sex Diaries Project* for this reason—it shows in a pretty clear light what regular people think about their sex lives. Dan Savage's syndicated column *Savage Love* serves a similarly great purpose. Reading through those columns always makes me feel like I'm one of thousands of people who are just figuring out how to live the lives we want.

Finally, I love Cheryl Strayed's advice column collection *Tiny Beautiful Things*, which reinforces the idea of beginning the work of making better relationships by learning how to love yourself. Her writing sticks with me. Whenever I'm nervous to tell someone how much I like them, I'm reminded of her idea that love is like an iron bell and you should ring it every chance you get.

THANK YOU
Oh geez.

This book is a community project. I am honored that so many friends and strangers trusted me enough to talk about the scariest parts of themselves. Thank you so much to every person who spoke with me about their relationships—this book is for you and I hope it does justice to the bravery you all showed in being up for digging deep with me.

Thank you to my long-time-romantic-partner and now-good-friend Carl, who always pushes me to be more honest and who is the smartest person in the universe.

Thank you to my family. Everyone in the world deserves parents as thoughtful, as fair, and as supportive as my parents. Also thanks to my brother, who is a jerk. Just kidding. Thanks for never letting me take myself too seriously, Dan.

Thank you to my supportive coworkers at the *Portland Mercury*, who for some reason let me leave work for three months to start this book. Thank you to my extremely generous and impressive coworkers at *Bitch* for creating a workplace where it's okay not to be okay all the time. Thank you for providing a place where I can do good work fighting the big scary stuff and, on a personal level, for knowing when I desperately need some hot chocolate.

Thank you to the friends who read drafts of these chapters and gave me feedback: Carl, Travis, Kate, Ledah, and Grant. Tremendous thanks to the people I've dated over the years—especially Anand and Cyrus—for being wonderful and for bearing with me as I've figured myself out.

Thanks to Microcosm for publishing this book! Thanks to Natalie Nourigat and Molly Schaeffer for their wonderful illustrations. Thanks to the folks who hang out at Portland's Independent Publishing Resource Center for helping me see myself as someone with ideas worth sharing. Thanks to The Waypost, where I wrote most of this book and where the bartenders are always kind.

Finally, I have immense, overwhelming, heart-wrenching gratitude for my friends, who always surprise me with their deep love and good ideas. Thank you to the friends-for-life in Portland, Seattle, LA, San Francisco, Oakland, New York, Vancouver, Chicago, Madison, and Boston who let me sleep on their sofas while researching and writing this book. They were all very nice sofas. Your names would take up three pages so I won't list them all out but thank you, thank you, friends all over, for your support and for your enduring humor in the face of bullshit.

MOST IMPORTANT NEEDS
FOR MY PARTNER:

- **SUPPORT AND APPRECIATION OF ME:** They've got to understand who I am, respect me & my work, and help me feel good about myself. ‥⌣

- **LOVE THEMSELVES:** They need to feel confident about who they are & have an independent life & interests they're excited about. Help expand my world!

- **CURIOSITY ABOUT THE WORLD:** They need to have a desire to explore and learn new things together.

- **WE HAVE TO TALK** — We need to have communication that helps us feel better, not worse, & to draw each other out.

- **A SENSE OF HUMOR!** We have to be able to laugh when things go wrong.

- **BODY POSITIVE & SEXUAL SPARK** — We have to feel physically comfortable together and to want to have sex with each other

- **SIMILAR MORAL OUTLOOK:** They've got to recognize privilege and not be dogmatic.

NOT ABSOLUTELY NECESSARY (BUT STILL IMPORTANT) NEEDS:

- SELF-SUPPORTING: They've got to be able to take care of their finances and their body's health.
- PRIORITIZE GOOD FRIENDSHIPS: They need to have people they talk and connect with (and spend time with) besides me.
- LIKES TO BE BUSY: I've got a million events and meetings, he could get overwhelmed.
- POLITICALLY ENGAGED: Agh. What if he doesn't vote??

NEEDS I'M NOT SURE ABOUT:

- Kids??
- Lives in Portland
- Age...?

SUBSCRIBE TO EVERYTHING WE PUBLISH!

Do you love what Microcosm publishes?

Do you want us to publish more great stuff?

Would you like to receive each new title as it's published?

Subscribe as a BFF to our new titles and we'll mail them all to you as they are released!

$10-30/mo, pay what you can afford. Include your t-shirt size and month/date of birthday for a possible surprise! Subscription begins the month after it is purchased.

microcosmpublishing.com/bff

...AND HELP US GROW YOUR SMALL WORLD!